Your Child's Best Shot

A parent's guide to vaccination

2nd edition

Ronald Gold, MD, MPH

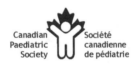

Canadian
Paediatric
Society

Société
canadienne
de pédiatrie

Copyright © Canadian Paediatric Society, 2002
ISBN 0-9682409-6-8 (English paperback)
ISBN 0-9682409-7-6 (French paperback)

Printed and bound in Canada

Canadian Cataloguing-in-Publication Data

Your child's best shot: a parent's guide to vaccination. — 2nd ed.

Includes bibliographical references and index.
ISBN 0-9682409-6-8

1. Vaccination of children—Popular works. 2. Vaccines—Popular works. 3. Communicable diseases—Popular works. I. Canadian Paediatric Society

RJ240.Y68 2002   614.4'7'083   C2002-904001-9

This title is available in English and French, and may be ordered from the:

Canadian Paediatric Society
100-2204 Walkley Road
Ottawa ON K1G 4G8
Tel. (613)526-9397
Fax. (613)526-3332
<www.cps.ca>

Cover and book design: Fairmont House Design
Editing: Mary Jean McAleer and Shelley Henderson
Cover image: (detail) Miranda Angel, St. Elias Community School, Haines Junction, Yukon Territory
Translation: Dominique Paré (Le bout de la langue)

The publisher gives permission to health care professionals to reproduce the fact sheets and tables in Chapter 19 and share them with patients and their families.

Contents

Tables

Acknowledgements

The second edition of *Your Child's Best Shot: A Parent's Guide to Vaccination* was reviewed by the Canadian Paediatric Society's 2001–02 Infectious Diseases and Immunization Committee:

Members
Joanne E. Embree, MD (Chair), Department of Pediatrics and Child Health and the Department of Medical Microbiology, University of Manitoba, Winnipeg, Manitoba

Gary Pekeles, MD, Director, Northern Health Program, Montreal Children's Hospital, McGill University Health Centre, and Associate Professor, Department of Pediatrics, McGill University, Montreal, Quebec

Upton Dilworth Allen, MD, Associate Professor of Pediatrics, Division of Infectious Diseases, Hospital for Sick Children, University of Toronto, Toronto, Ontario

H. Dele Davies, MD, Division of Infectious Diseases, Alberta Children's Hospital, Calgary, Alberta

Joanne M. Langley, MD, Department of Pediatrics, Dalhousie University, Clinical Trials Research Centre, IWK Health Centre, Halifax, Nova Scotia

Mireille D. Lemay, MD, Department of Infectious Diseases, Hôpital Sainte-Justine, Montreal, Quebec

Liaisons
Scott Alan Halperin, MD, IMPACT (Immunization Monitoring Program ACTive), Clinical Trials Research Centre, Dalhousie University and IWK Centre, Halifax, Nova Scotia

Susan M. King, MD, Division of Infectious Diseases, Hospital for Sick Children, University of Toronto, Toronto, Ontario

Monique Landry, MD, Medical Officer, Public Health Division, ministère de la Santé et des Services sociaux, Montreal, Québec

Larry Pickering, MD, FAAP, Editor, *Red Book*, Committee on Infectious Diseases, American Academy of Pediatrics, Atlanta, Georgia

Consultants
Gilles Delage, MD, Senior Director, Medical Affairs, Héma-Québec, St-Laurent, Quebec

Noni MacDonald, MD, Department of Paediatrics, Division of Infectious Diseases, Dalhousie University, Halifax, Nova Scotia

Victor Marchessault, MD, Professor of Pediatrics and Infectious Diseases, Children's Hospital of Eastern Ontario, Ottawa, Ontario

Principal Author
Ronald Gold, MD, Honorary Consultant, Division of Infectious Diseases, Hospital for Sick Children; Professor Emeritus of Pediatrics, University of Toronto, Toronto, Ontario

The Canadian Paediatric Society wishes to acknowledge the following corporate sponsors for their unrestricted educational grants in support of this publication:

Aventis Pasteur Limited
GlaxoSmithKline
Merck Frosst Canada Inc.
Wyeth-Ayerst Canada Inc.

The Canadian Paediatric Society gratefully acknowledges the generous support of the Division of Immunization and Respiratory Diseases, Centre for Infectious Disease Prevention and Control, Population and Public Health Branch, Health Canada. We also wish to acknowledge the contribution of the British Columbia Ministry of Health and Ministry Responsible for Seniors, as well as the Ontario Ministry of Health and Long-Term Care.

Special thanks are due to Drs. Danielle Grenier and Claude Paré for their careful review of this book.

Our thanks to the many Grade 6 Canadian children who took part in the National Immunization Poster Competition in 2000. Selections of their artwork appear throughout this book.

Foreword

Nowadays, parents often worry more about how their children will react to their immunization shots than about the risk of their children catching the diseases against which they are being immunized. Will vaccination hurt? Will my child have a bad reaction?

Not so many years ago, it was the other way around: parents worried far more about the diseases than about the vaccines. And it's not hard to understand why this reversal has occurred. After all, parents today no longer hear about friends' or relatives' children becoming paralyzed by polio, or dying of diphtheria or tetanus (lockjaw). Even the most common form of childhood meningitis — which caused many deaths and much permanent disability just a few years ago — has almost disappeared because of vaccination.

Childhood immunization has saved millions of lives by eliminating many serious childhood diseases. This truth is undisputable. But by virtue of its very effectiveness, immunization has come under scrutiny and has sometimes been deemed unnecessary and even harmful. The media's focus on these aspects of vaccination combined with the reality that we no longer hear about many of these diseases in our own communities leads some parents to develop a false sense of security. They can easily become complacent about the need to have their children fully protected and about the importance of keeping immunizations up to date.

But the fact is that in recent years, several countries have experienced new outbreaks of diseases that everyone thought had disappeared — like diphtheria, German measles (rubella) and polio. These diseases reappeared either because governments had relaxed their immunization programs or because certain groups in the population had refused immunizations for their children, for religious or other reasons. The danger of inadequate immunization never disappears.

Those of us who remember the thousands of Canadian children stricken with polio or meningitis and the deaths and permanent damage inflicted by those diseases appreciate the miracles that have been achieved by vaccines that are now available to everyone.

There is no doubt that miracles of disease prevention lie ahead as new vaccines are developed. Researchers are constantly testing new combinations of vaccines designed to give children maximum protection with as few injections as possible. In addition, various methods are now being used to make injections less painful. Thanks to today's vaccines and to other advances in child health care, fewer children are being hospitalized than ever before.

So, every parent should be aware that diseases like polio, diphtheria, rubella, *Haemophilus influenzae* type b, meningitis and hepatitis B *can* and *will* reappear if we become complacent or forgetful about having our children fully protected through immunization. Even the best-intentioned parents can forget which shots their children have received or when they are due for booster shots. Therefore all parents should keep a written record of their children's immunizations. Your doctor or the Canadian Paediatric Society can provide you with a special booklet for this purpose.

Parents should also be aware that there is a lot of scary misinformation being circulated about vaccines and their supposed risks. The source of much of this misinformation and rumour-mongering is the Internet. This new and wonderful technology offers great opportunity to those who want to share information. Unfortunately, not all information can be trusted!

The saying "you can't believe everything you read" most certainly holds true for the subject of vaccination. The authenticity of many information sources is questionable. Individuals and organizations with authoritative-sounding titles spout all kinds of horror stories, statistics and warnings; however they do not represent authoritative or reliable sources.

If you have questions or doubts about the information you read or hear, you can always rely on organizations like the Canadian Paediatric Society to give you thoroughly dependable, up-to-date information and advice, based on solid, scientific evidence. Your paediatrician, family doctor, or public health nurse can also provide you with recent and reliable information as well as suggest reputable sources and websites.

This book gives you the most current information on all aspects of vaccination. The fact that you are reading this book indicates that you want your child to be safe and protected against serious communicable diseases. I applaud you for doing your homework and researching the issue. But please consult only reliable sources. Ask your trusted physician/paediatrician any questions you have about vaccination. If you follow the guidelines in this book, you can rest assured knowing that you have given your children your best shot.

Richard Goldbloom, MD, O.C.
Professor of Paediatrics
Dalhousie University
Halifax, Nova Scotia

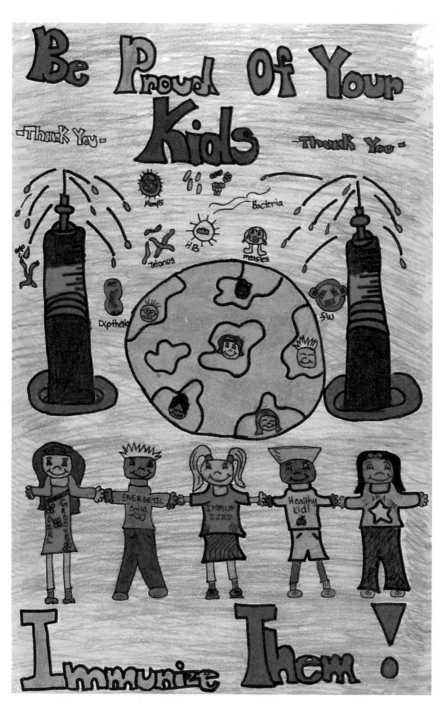

April Miranda, Winnipeg, Manitoba

Introduction

There are many reasons why people will read this book. Some parents are in favour of vaccination but just want to learn more. Some have heard scary stories and want to see what more they can find out. Others are unsure about the need for vaccines in today's world.

There is only one reason this book was written: to inform people about vaccination — with truthful, current, complete and understandable information.

A Wealth of Misinformation

Parents who are trying to educate themselves about vaccine safety will have no problem finding information. The difficulty lies in trying to figure out which information to believe, especially when every article, website and "official report" has a new angle. The media focus on the most headline-grabbing stories — often they feature alarmists who make unfounded claims, propose unsupported theories and cite false statistics.

I sympathize with parents who, in their search for the truth, come across this type of material. One cannot help but wonder what is fact and what is fiction. The purpose of becoming knowledgeable on the subject of vaccines is to help your child obtain the proper health care. To achieve this goal, your decisions must be based on facts, meaning information that comes from reliable authors and sources.

Getting the Facts Straight

Immunization of children is one of the most important aspects of maintaining their health. Before many of today's vaccines were available, it was not uncommon for children to die or become disabled as a result of infections that are now preventable. The following question illustrates a common myth and may help you understand how making a decision based on misinformation could prove harmful for your family.

I recently heard that if I decide not to vaccinate my children, they will be protected from diseases anyway because everyone else is vaccinated. Is this true?

No. This approach doesn't work, for one reason — you cannot always control your environment, including the people around you and the air you breathe. Disease can spread through travel and via the environment.

Spread via travel. People who travel are at risk of being exposed to infections that have become rare in Canada, but still thrive in other places. In recent years, Russia, the Ukraine, the Netherlands, England, Japan and Sweden have experienced new outbreaks of diseases that everyone thought had disappeared — diphtheria, German measles (rubella) and polio. These diseases reappeared either because governments had relaxed their immunization programs or because certain members of the population had refused immunization for their children for their own reasons.

Partial immunization is like partial fumigation — sterilizing every room in a house but one. The bugs in that room will multiply and spread throughout the house. Similarly, diseases *can* and *will* reappear if children are not fully protected through immunization.

Although these countries are far away from North America, with travel being as frequent as it is these days, it does not take long for disease to be brought into Canada and affect our children.

Spread via environment. Tetanus (lockjaw) is different from other vaccine-preventable diseases because you get it from the environment, not from other persons. Tetanus bacteria form spores (capsules), allowing the bacteria to survive in the soil as well as in dust inside houses and hospitals. These spores are highly resistant to heat and ultraviolet light, which allows the bacteria to survive many years outside the body.

When dirt that contains spores gets into a cut or wound, the bacteria in the spores grow and produce the toxin (poison) that causes tetanus. Vaccination is the most effective way to prevent this disease.

Nowhere to hide. Without question, the germs will "find" people who are susceptible (not protected). You may think that your children will "get lost in the crowd," or that your children have no contact with world travellers and therefore are not at risk.

But what if your neighbours return after being posted in a developing country for a few years and your children want to play with their old friends? Families come to Canada from countries all over the world. Can you prevent contact between your children and others who may not be vaccinated — at school? at the mall? at a birthday party? As for tetanus, will your children never play outdoors? Even if you kept your children indoors, you could not protect them from this disease. Tetanus spores are so common, they can even be found in the dust in hospitals! They will most certainly be living in household dust.

Clearly, germs can invade your children's environment in countless ways. You can't hide from the germs, but you *can* protect your children through vaccination.

Information You Can Trust

Children are precious; their health and well-being mean everything. They depend on you to make decisions for them every day, and this

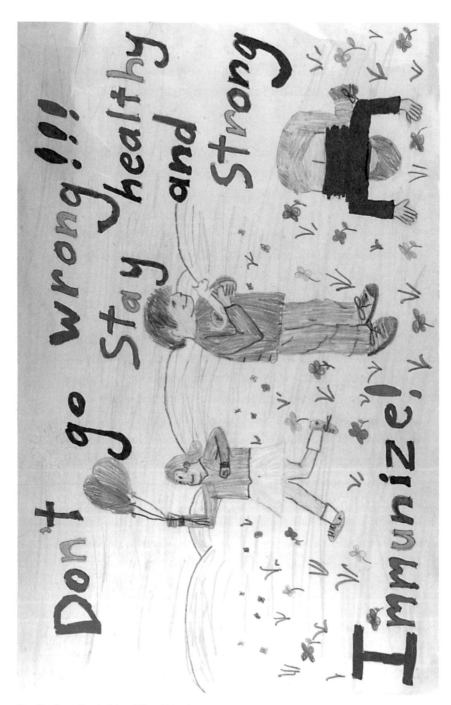

Troy Dearborn, Souris, Prince Edward Island

is a big one. You can't make a decision about vaccination without proper information. You need to know the facts about vaccines *and* disease.

Here, in one book, you'll find important information on childhood infections. Chapters 1 and 2 lay the groundwork for understanding all of the chapters that follow. Chapter 1 explains how the immune system works. It is important to understand this to know how infection and vaccines create immunity to disease. Chapter 2 describes the medical system that monitors the safety and effectiveness of vaccines. Don't skip over these chapters — they contain important information that you should know.

Chapters 3 to 15 provide complete descriptions of illnesses for which there is a vaccine. You'll find everything you want — and need — to know about each illness and the corresponding vaccine. Chapter 16 deals with vaccines that are used mainly for people travelling abroad. If you have further questions, check Chapter 17. It answers 32 common questions that parents ask about vaccination.

Chapter 18 provides advice on assessing information about vaccines. To help you with your research on the subject of vaccination, several trustworthy websites and other resources have been listed and described at the end of the chapter. For quick reference, a series of fact sheets have been prepared that provide basic information about diseases and vaccines. These appear in Chapter 19, along with a recommended schedule of childhood vaccination.

Easy Reading

This book contains scientific material, so you may come across some unfamiliar terms. However, this book was written for parents, not doctors and scientists. Terms have been explained using familiar language wherever possible. If you have questions, please contact the Canadian Paediatric Society. You'll find contact information at the beginning of this book.

Whatever reason has led you to pick up this book, you'll be glad you did. It contains information that will benefit our most precious asset — our children and youth.

Douglas D. McMillan, MD, FRCPC
President, Canadian Paediatric Society
2002–03

CHAPTER 1

How Vaccines Work

Most parents wonder how a needle filled with fluid keeps their child safe from disease. The purpose of this chapter is to help you understand how vaccines work.

The goal of a vaccine is to make a person immune to a germ. To understand how this is possible, you first have to know how the immune system works.

The Immune System

The immune system is a complex of special cells and proteins that move through the body to protect it against infection. The immune system is designed to identify and remove foreign substances (such as germs) from the body. The germs causing the diseases described in this book are either bacteria or viruses.

Germs

Bacteria are microscopic organisms. They are "complete" in that they are able to live on their own as long as they have essential chemicals to nourish them.

Viruses, on the other hand, are "incomplete" organisms; they are unable to live on their own. To grow and reproduce, the virus must get inside a cell. Once inside, the virus takes over the function of the cell and uses it to make new virus particles.

Bacteria and viruses have unique proteins and polysaccharides (complex sugars) on their surfaces called *antigens*. They are very different from human proteins and sugars. Some surface antigens allow the germ to stick to human cells (this is the first step of infection). Others protect the germ against the body's defences. The immune system targets these antigens.

The Body's Defences

The immune system responds to bacteria and viruses in a very complex way: it produces **antibodies** (a type of protein) and special white blood cells called **lymphocytes**. Both antibodies and lymphocytes work by combining with or attaching to an antigen on the surface of a bacterium or virus.

Antibodies. When antibodies attach to a bacterium or virus, it is much easier for the white blood cells to take over and destroy the germ. The immune system can also make specific antibodies that latch onto toxins (poisons) produced by germs. Antibodies block the action of the toxin and make it easier for the body to get rid of the toxin.

Lymphocytes. These special white blood cells are the backbone of the immune system. Some, called B-lymphocytes or *B-cells*, make antibodies. Others, called T-lymphocytes or *T-cells*, have a number of different jobs. For example, they help the immune system identify the presence of germs such as bacteria and viruses. They also stimulate the B-cells to grow, divide and produce antibodies. Some T-cells can even recognize cells that are infected with a virus and kill both the infected cell and the virus.

Memory cells are also very important lymphocytes. They live a very long time, if not for life. Therefore, memory cells enable the immune system to recognize germs it has seen before — even many years before — so that it can kill the germs before any damage occurs.

Immunity

Immune Memory

Memory cells create a very strong memory (called **immune memory**) for the immune system. Once the immune system has "seen" a certain germ (meaning it has been stimulated by that germ), it will be able to recognize it again very quickly and act on it for a very long time. Long-lasting immunity to infection depends on the immune memory cells.

It is important to understand that *immune memory is very specific*. Each germ triggers a unique response in the immune system. A specific set of T-cells, B-cells and memory cells are programmed to detect and react to one, and only one, germ.

When the immune system has acquired the ability to rapidly identify the presence of a specific germ and destroy it before it causes damage, **immunity** to that germ has been established.

Achieving Immunity

Two ways. Now that you know how the immune system works, you may be wondering what the difference is between immunity achieved by *natural infection* and by *vaccine*. (A vaccine is a substance that stimulates [or induces] the immune system to make antibodies, T-cells and memory cells — the body's main defences against infection.) To illustrate the difference, let's use measles as an example.

Natural infection. The first time a person is exposed to the natural form of the measles virus (i.e., by airborne particles), the virus infects many cells and causes illness before the immune response has developed. Infection from measles can do a lot of damage. (In severe cases, the infection spreads so rapidly that the person dies before immunity can be established.) Once a person has had measles, immune memory is established and the person is immune to the virus.

Vaccine. After the measles vaccine is injected into a person, it stimulates antibodies and lymphocytes (including memory cells), creating immune memory. The person may have a little redness and swelling at the injection site. Vaccination with measles vaccine establishes long-lasting immunity to measles.

Are they the same kind of immunity? Yes. Although there are two ways of achieving immunity, the end result is the same. In both examples above (natural infection and vaccine), the person becomes immune to measles virus. The next time the person is exposed to the measles virus, the immune system responds so quickly that the virus is destroyed before it can cause an infection.

So what's the difference? The person who had the vaccine did not endure the illness and its potentially life-threatening complications.

Vaccines

Types of Vaccines

Immunization (or vaccination) is a method of providing protection against disease caused by infection. Just as there are several different types of infections, there are several types of vaccines [see Table 1.1 below].

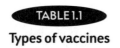
TABLE 1.1

Types of vaccines

TYPE OF VACCINE	EXAMPLES
Killed, intact bacteria	Typhoid vaccine
Killed, intact virus	Inactivated polio vaccine, hepatitis A vaccine
Killed, disrupted virus	Influenza vaccine
Live, weakened or attenuated bacteria	Oral typhoid vaccine
Live, weakened or attenuated virus	Oral polio, measles, mumps, rubella and chickenpox vaccines
Purified bacterial proteins	Acellular pertussis vaccine
Purified bacterial polysaccharide or complex sugar	*Haemophilus influenzae* type b, pneumococcal and meningococcal vaccines
Purified viral protein	Hepatitis B vaccine
Inactivated bacterial toxin	Diphtheria and tetanus toxoids

This Table was not put here to scare you away! Yes, it contains a lot of long and unfamiliar terms. But throughout the book, each term will be explained.

From the Table, you can see that not all vaccines are the same type. They differ in many ways: what's in them, how they are made and stored, and how they are given to children, to name just a few. They don't differ, though, in their purpose or in the way they are tested. (Vaccine testing will be covered in the next chapter.)

The Purpose of Vaccines

Immunity. Modern vaccines are designed to prevent disease by producing immune responses without the risk of illness or death associated with the infection. The principle of vaccination is simple: exposing the immune system to a vaccine containing germs or parts of germs causes the immune system to respond just as it does to the actual infection.

Controlled exposure to germ. Scientists know that the body makes the same antibodies and T-cells that it would in response to an infection. They also know that introducing the immune system to germs creates the all-important immune memory. The key advantage of creating immune memory via vaccine is that the amount of exposure to the germ is controlled. Immune memory can be established without the threat of serious illness from an uncontrolled infection.

Side Effects of Vaccines

The risks of side effects caused by vaccines are well known and documented, as are the risks of illness and complications caused by natural infection. The risks associated with vaccines are far fewer and far less severe than those associated with disease.

Most parents know that vaccines are tested before they can be used on the public. But they don't know the extent of monitoring, testing, information sharing and decision making that goes on behind the scenes. All year round, year after year, a network of professionals, committees and organizations keeps a watchful eye on reported side effects and reactions following vaccination. The next chapter describes the systems that are in place to ensure the safety of vaccines.

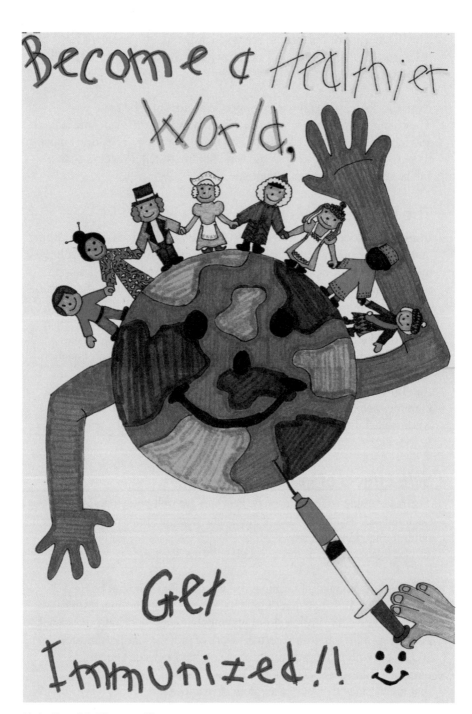

Kaylee Kostyniuk, Edmonton, Alberta

CHAPTER 2

Vaccine Safety, Testing and Effectiveness

The first part of this chapter discusses the large network of professionals, committees and organizations that oversees diseases and vaccines. Their role is to monitor safety, testing and effectiveness of vaccines and make recommendations based on their knowledge of diseases and vaccines. Unlike some sources of information available today, these experts can be trusted to provide sound decisions based on the most up-to-date and credible information.

The second part describes the methods used by scientists to test vaccines for safety (e.g., are there any side effects?) and effectiveness (e.g., do the vaccines do what they are supposed to?) and to determine whether claims (of any severity) against vaccines are true.

Vaccine Safety

Vaccines, like all medicines, must go through a series of steps before they are approved for use. Health authorities in Canada, including those in provincial and federal governments and the Canadian Paediatric Society, take vaccine safety very seriously. Before any vaccine is approved for use in Canada, it must be shown to be safe and effective in preventing the disease that it targets.

The **Bureau of Biologics and Radiopharmaceuticals (BOBR)**, which is part of Health Canada, regulates vaccines used in humans in Canada. Vaccines are licensed by the BOBR for use in Canada only if they meet acceptable standards of production, safety and potency. All batches of vaccine must pass the safety and potency tests before they are released for use.

Production. The BOBR supervises all aspects of vaccine production by the manufacturers. Before any vaccine is licensed and approved for use in Canada, the factory where it is manufactured must be inspected to ensure that all stages of production meet the requirements for safety, sterility and quality control.

Safety. The BOBR decides which tests must be performed to evaluate the safety of each batch of vaccine. Most safety tests are carried out by both the manufacturer and the laboratory of the BOBR.

Potency. Potency tests of each batch of vaccine are also specified by the BOBR. (Potency refers to the efficacy of a vaccine, meaning its ability to induce the desired response by the immune system.)

Monitoring Vaccine Safety

Canada has systems to monitor the safety of vaccines that have been approved by the BOBR. Today, Canada is a world leader in "post-marketing surveillance of vaccine adverse events." This means that medical experts in Canada are made aware of unusual post-vaccine events.

One way the information gets passed to Health Canada is through **health officials:**

- In all provinces, doctors and public health nurses report to the local health department any adverse events and local and general reactions that occur after vaccination. (Adverse events are more severe than local or general reactions, which include soreness, redness, swelling or fever.)
- The local medical officer of health investigates these reports, then forwards them to the provincial ministry of health.
- The reports then go to the Division of Immunization, Centre for Infectious Disease Prevention and Control, Health Canada. This federal agency keeps track of and analyzes all of the reports of adverse events after vaccination. The division receives about 4,000 reports each year. Most reports concern minor events such as fever or local reactions.

IMPACT. Canada has a unique program, called IMPACT, to detect severe adverse events related to vaccination. IMPACT stands for **I**mmunization **M**onitoring **P**rogram, **ACT**ive. The program is funded by the Division of Immunization, Centre for Infectious Disease Prevention and Control, Health Canada, and is operated by the Canadian Paediatric Society.

IMPACT was designed by researchers at paediatric centres in Canada who were interested in vaccination. The program works as follows:

- A nurse at each of 12 children's hospitals across Canada reviews all admissions to the hospital for certain serious illnesses such as seizures, encephalitis, encephalopathy and acute paralysis. Each year, these nurses screen more than 90,000 children admitted to the 12 hospitals.
- In their reports, the nurses record specifics about the illness and get a detailed immunization history from the parents, family doctor or immunization clinic to determine whether the illness happened after vaccination.
- The reports are sent to the IMPACT data centre for analysis. The Division of Immunization receives monthly reports. Detailed annual

reports are examined by the Infectious Diseases and Immunization Committee of the Canadian Paediatric Society [see next section for further information on this committee]. The information acquired by IMPACT is also published in medical journals.

IMPACT has been running since 1991 and has confirmed that severe neurologic illness occurring after vaccination is extremely rare. Athough seizures following vaccination have been reported, no cases of encephalitis, encephalopathy or acute paralysis have been linked to vaccination.

With the **Canadian Paediatric Surveillance Program (CPSP)**, Canada has another valuable and unique surveillance tool for collecting active real-time data on rare diseases, including vaccine-preventable diseases.

Established through a partnership between Health Canada's Centre for Infectious Disease Prevention and Control and the Canadian Paediatric Society, the CPSP has been in operation since 1996. The program involves more than 2,350 paediatricians and paediatric subspecialists from all provinces and territories, who monitor their practices for rare conditions and report monthly to the CPSP.

Through the years, this program has collected much needed data on the efficacy and safety of vaccines and on the rarity of vaccine-preventable diseases and their consequences, such as congenital rubella syndrome, necrotizing fasciitis (a serious infection arising from chickenpox) and subacute sclerosing panencephalitis (a serious complication of measles).

In addition, CPSP surveillance of acute flaccid paralysis enabled Canada to fulfill its international obligations to the Pan American Health Organization and the World Health Organization by demonstrating the absence of paralytic polio and wild polioviruses in Canada.

Advisory Committee on Causality Assessment. This committee reviews all reported cases of severe adverse events that occur following vaccination. Members include experts in paediatrics, public health, epidemiology (the study of diseases to learn about incidence, control and prevention), infectious diseases, immunology and neurology.

The committee meets four days a year to review the severe or unexpected adverse events after vaccination that were reported to either the Division of Immunization or IMPACT. Included in the review are all cases of meningitis/encephalitis, encephalopathy, seizures without fever, death or any event that required hospitalization following immunization. Because most such events are not caused by vaccination but are linked by coincidence, it is important to review the details of all cases.

The purpose of the Advisory Committee is to determine whether the adverse event and the implicated vaccine are:
• related;
• possibly related;
• unlikely to have been related;
• unrelated.

Based on its review, the committee can recommend that regulatory action be considered (i.e., that the federal government consider changes regarding licensing of the vaccine) or that further research be undertaken.

The committee reports the results of its reviews to the doctor or nurse reporting the event, Health Canada's Division of Immunization, IMPACT, and the Infectious Diseases and Immunization Committee of the Canadian Paediatric Society. The Advisory Committee on Causality Assessment also publishes reports of its reviews in medical journals.

Immunization Safety Review Committee. The Institute of Medicine (IOM) in the United States formed this committee to evaluate the available evidence on various immunization safety concerns. Specifically, the committee was asked to present their findings regarding possible causal associations between vaccines and certain adverse outcomes. The committee meets whenever issues concerning vaccines are identified.

The Immunization Safety Review Committee includes experts in infectious diseases, immunization, epidemiology, statistics and public health. It does an extensive review of relevant published scientific and medical articles as well as unpublished data, personal communications, and submissions by any interested parties. The committee's conclusions and recommendations (listed below) are published by the National Academy of Sciences. They are also available from the IOM's website (www.iom.edu/iom/iomhome.nsf/Pages/immunization+safety+review):

- *Adverse Effects Following Pertussis and Rubella Vaccines* (1991);
- *Adverse Events Associated with Childhood Vaccines: Evidence Bearing on Causality* (1994);
- *DTaP Vaccine and Chronic Nervous System Dysfunction: A New Analysis* (1994);
- *Immunization Safety Review: Measles-Mumps-Rubella Vaccine and Autism* (2001);
- *Immunization Safety Review: Thimerosal-Containing Vaccines and Neurodevelopmental Disorders* (2001).

Making Recommendations on Vaccine Use

NACI. The National Advisory Committee on Immunization (NACI) reviews all of the information obtained from the sources discussed above as well as from the Infectious Diseases and Immunization Committee, and makes recommendations on the use of vaccines in Canada. The NACI recommendations are used by the ministries of health in each of the provinces and territories to develop their immunization programs.

This committee reports to the federal minister of health. It includes non-governmental experts in infectious diseases, immunization, immunology, epidemiology and public health.
- The committee regularly reviews all the scientific information available on the safety and efficacy of vaccines and publishes its recommendations on vaccine use in the *Canadian Communicable Disease Report.*

- It issues updated statements on vaccine safety whenever appropriate.
- The committee also publishes the *Canadian Immunization Guide* every four years, which contains all of the current recommendations. All doctors and public health agencies in Canada receive copies of the guide.
- NACI also exchanges information with the U.S. Public Health Service. The NACI chairman is a member of the U.S. Public Service's Advisory Committee on Immunization Practices (ACIP) and attends all of the meetings of that committee as well. A member of ACIP also attends NACI meetings. This two-way liaison between the Canadian and American committees ensures that members of the committee in Canada are up-to-date with recommendations made by the committee in the United States, as well as with the information that they base their decisions on.

Infectious Diseases and Immunization Committee. This committee is part of the Canadian Paediatric Society and it also makes recommendations about vaccines and immunization programs. Many members of this committee are also members of NACI. The chairperson of the committee acts as a liaison with the Committee on Infectious Diseases of the American Academy of Pediatrics. This person attends all meetings of both committees and participates in writing the American recommendations on vaccine use.

These recommendations are published in *Paediatrics & Child Health*, the journal of the Canadian Paediatric Society, in *Pediatrics*, the journal of the American Academy of Pediatrics, and in the *Report of the Committee*, called the *Red Book* (because of the colour of its cover). The *Red Book* is published every three years. It contains information on vaccination and infectious diseases in children. The editor of the *Red Book* is a liaison member of the Infectious Diseases and Immunization Committee in Canada.

Keeping up-to-date. With so much crossover among these committees, all members — Canadian and American alike — are up-to-date with vaccine policies and recommendations in both countries.

Testing Vaccine Safety and Effectiveness

The Science of Cause and Effect

How do scientists determine whether a vaccine causes an adverse event? And how do they determine whether a vaccine prevents disease? The same principles are used to answer both questions. Since parents are most often concerned about the safety of vaccines, the following discussion explains how scientists use different methods to try to answer questions about causes of adverse events seen after vaccination. A simple example has been used to illustrate the different methods.

Temporal vs. causal association. One event, for example, eating ice cream (event A) may be followed by another event, such as sweating (event B). Events that occur in this way are said to be temporally associated — related to each other in time. This doesn't necessarily mean there is a cause and effect relationship. In other words, the fact that event B follows event A does not mean that A caused B; it may just be a coincidence.

Proof vs. probability. Science cannot prove that one event can *never* cause another. For instance, it cannot prove that eating ice cream (event A) will never make a person sweat (event B). What science *can* determine is the probability of these events happening. For example, it can determine the *likelihood* that eating ice cream will make a person sweat. Or, to be more exact, science can determine the probability of a particular outcome having occurred by chance.

Everyday example. Imagine that a person did sweat after eating ice cream. Scientists could review all of the circumstances surrounding the event and tell us their findings: it is 99.9% certain that these two events happened by chance — it was the extreme heat that day that made the person sweat, not the ice cream. In this case, the events of eating the ice cream and sweating are linked in time: there is a temporal association. There is no causal association.

A vaccine-related example. If the probability is high that chance could lead to an association between events A and B, then we cannot conclude that A caused B. For example, a small proportion of babies who have died of sudden infant death syndrome (SIDS) had been vaccinated within a day of dying. Did vaccination cause the death? Many studies have shown that there is no increased risk of SIDS following vaccination. The association between vaccination and SIDS is purely coincidental. It occurs because vaccination is very common between two and six months of age, the time period when most cases of SIDS occur.

But, the association between a baby's sleeping position (event A) and SIDS (event B) has been found to be causal: event A causes event B. Babies who sleep on their stomachs are much more likely to die of SIDS than babies who sleep on their backs. Results of the "Back to Sleep" campaign, which was designed to raise awareness about the back-sleep position, confirm the causal association between sleep position and SIDS:

- More than two-thirds of parents put their babies on their back to sleep in Canada and the United States.
- Since this change, the occurrence rate of SIDS has been cut almost in half in Canada, the United States, New Zealand and many other countries.

Analyzing Data

How scientists determine the type of association. By examining several different kinds of information, scientists can learn whether one event causes another. Once they have analyzed existing data and have performed experiments of their own, they use the seven criteria discussed below to help determine whether the two events they are working with (A and B) are associated and if so, how. (Not all of the criteria apply in every situation.)

Let's use the ice cream and sweating example again.

1. *Unique and specific outcome.* Is the outcome, or event B (for example, sweating), a unique and specific reaction that occurs only

after the introduction of the cause in question (event A, eating ice cream) and never at other times?

2. **Unique and specific pathology.** Does event B involve unique and specific behaviour that occurs only after event A and never at other times? For example, is there anything unusual about the sweating that happens only after the person eats ice cream?

3. **Positive association in animal experimentation.** Does event A produce event B in animals in controlled experiments? For example, do animals sweat after eating ice cream in a laboratory?

4. **Close temporal association.** Do the two events happen within the same time period? A temporal association is a necessary condition of cause and effect. But it is not sufficient proof that one causes the other, since the temporal association could be purely coincidental (as explained in the SIDS example, above). To learn whether event B occurs after event A, careful investigation of a number of cases of event B is carried out.

   In our ice cream example, scientists would review other cases that involved eating ice cream and sweating. (Other reasons for the sweating could be nervousness, a medical condition involving the sweat glands, or eating while sitting beside a roaring fire.)

5. **Demonstrable biological mechanism.** The process by which event A produces event B should be able to be explained by information that is credible and known to be true (e.g., the laws of physics, the digestive system). In the example being used, researchers would have to find a biological explanation for the ice cream causing a person to sweat.

6. **Positive relationship regarding frequency of events.** One of the main methods of gathering and testing information in epidemiology (the study of diseases to learn about incidence, control and prevention) is to study groups of people. Studies can show whether event A increases the frequency or risk of event B. In the example given, researchers would study groups of people eating ice cream to find

out how many, how often and under what circumstances people sweat while eating ice cream.

7. *Likelihood of coincidence.* Researchers and scientists also perform experimental studies. They compare two groups of subjects to find out the frequency or risk of event B (sweating) in both groups. The experimental group is exposed to event A (they eat ice cream), but the control group is not exposed (they don't eat ice cream). The frequency of event B in the two groups is compared and analyzed using statistical methods. From the results, researchers and scientists can determine the likelihood that the difference observed between the two groups is due to chance. If the likelihood is high, there is no casual association.

How many people would be sweating eating the ice cream? How many people not eating the ice cream would be sweating? The results would probably be the same in both groups.

Conclusion. When they had gathered all of the information available using the questions and methods above, scientists could conclude that there is a very, very low chance or probability that eating ice cream causes sweating.

Studying associations between vaccines and adverse outcomes. Epidemiologic studies (such as those described above) are frequently used to learn about associations between diseases and their suspected causes. Researchers and scientists use five special guidelines to help them analyze the results of such studies.

1. *Strength of association.* The strength of an association is measured in terms of relative risk. For example, let's use the frequency of sweating as our unit of measure. To calculate the relative risk between the sweating and eating ice cream, first, we tally the frequency of sweating occurring both in persons eating ice cream and in persons not eating ice cream. Then, we divide the rate in persons eating ice cream by the rate in persons not eating ice cream.

Relative risk equals 1.0. If the frequency is 2 (i.e., 2 people sweated while eating ice cream) for one group and 2 for the other group (i.e., 2 people sweated while not eating ice cream), the relative risk equals 1.0. In this case, there is no evidence of an increased risk in persons eating ice cream; there is no association between the ice cream and the sweating.

Relative risk greater than 1.0. If the relative risk is greater than 1.0 (i.e., 10 people sweated while eating ice cream but only 2 people sweated in the non-eating group), then there is evidence of a positive association. In this case, eating ice cream is likely causing the sweating. The greater the value of the relative risk, the greater the likelihood that the association is causal.

Relative risk less than 1.0. A relative risk of less than 1.0 (i.e., no one sweated while eating the ice cream but 4 people sweated in the non-eating group) means that there is no positive association; in this case, ice cream is very likely not causing the sweating.

2. **Dose-response relationship.** In a dose-response relationship, as the amount of ice cream eaten by a person increases, the risk of sweating also increases. However, the lack of a dose-response relationship does not rule out a causal relationship because a threshold may exist. In the example, this means that the sweating will occur, but not until a certain amount of ice cream has been eaten. For example, it may take 5 scoops of ice cream before a person starts to sweat. There is a dose-response relationship, but at a 5:1 ratio.

3. **Replication of findings.** If the association is causal, it should be found consistently in different studies.

4. **Alternative explanations.** A thorough search for all other causes or risk factors should be made in order to rule out alternative explanations.

5. **Cessation of exposure.** The frequency of event B (sweating) should decline on reduction or elimination of exposure to event A (eating ice cream).

Summary

A simple example — one that is unrelated to vaccines — has been used to make some of the points in this chapter clearer. These tests, studies and guidelines do apply to vaccines. Scientists and researchers use these same methods to make sure that vaccines are effective and safe. Based on all of the available scientific information, vaccines have been shown to be extremely effective and safe.

Vaccination has been and still is one of the most important means of preventing illness and disease. The benefits of vaccination far outweigh the extremely rare risks of serious adverse events.

Effectiveness of Vaccines

No vaccine is 100% effective, but all of the vaccines used for routine immunization of children are very effective in preventing disease. In fact, the vaccines are so effective that most of the diseases they protect against are now very rare.

Concerns About Side Effects

Most parents today have not had any direct experience with many of the infections described in this book, so they may not know about the serious and sometimes fatal outcomes of the diseases. As a result, some parents worry more about the side effects of vaccines than the diseases they prevent.

Although no vaccine is 100% safe, those described in this book carry an extremely low risk of serious side effects. The chapters that follow have been designed to bring parents up to speed on the vaccines *and* the diseases they protect against.

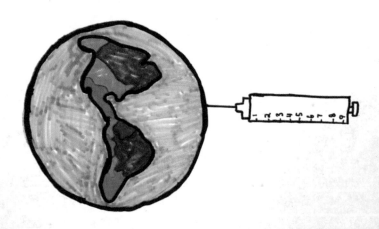

KEEP OUR WORLD HEALTHY!

Don't forget! BE IMMUNIZED!

Rylie Hamilton, Hay River, Northwest Territories

CHAPTER 3

Diphtheria

Diphtheria is an infection caused by bacteria called *Corynebacterium diphtheriae*. Diphtheria bacteria most often infect the nose or throat. Some strains make a toxin (poison) that can cause severe damage to the throat or other tissue. The toxin can attack the heart, nerves and kidneys as well. Diphtheria can also infect the skin.

The "D" in the combination DTaP vaccine stands for diphtheria.

A History of Diphtheria

Before Vaccine

Before 1900, diphtheria was one of the main causes of death of children. After 1900, improvements in social and economic conditions led to declining death rates for many common infections, including diphtheria. The death rate from diphtheria began to fall, but there was little change in the number of cases. Until 1920, approximately 12,000 cases and 1,000 deaths occurred every year in Canada.

Treatment for diphtheria first became available in the early 1920s, leading to further decline in death rates. Quarantine of cases was also introduced and rigidly enforced in major cities, which helped slow the spread of diphtheria.

After Vaccine

Diphtheria toxoid, the vaccine against diphtheria, was developed in the 1920s in France and Canada. Studies of children in Ontario between 1925 and 1930 found that the vaccine was highly effective. Routine immunization of children became widespread in Canada after 1930.

In 1924, 9,000 cases of diphtheria were reported in Canada. Since 1983, there have been fewer than 5 cases reported per year and no deaths. Diphtheria has become a very rare disease in all countries where children are immunized. Today, almost all cases of diphtheria in Canada and the United States occur in adults who have been either partially immunized or not immunized at all.

The Germ

How It Causes Illness

Diphtheria bacteria infect only humans. Most often, the bacteria infect the nose or throat. Much less frequently, they infect the skin.

Two forms of diphtheria bacteria occur: one produces toxin and the other does not. The bacteria release toxin as they grow and multiply, and the toxin causes the damage. If the infected person lacks protective antibodies, the toxin kills many of the cells lining the nose or throat.

The underlying tissues become red, swollen and painful. A thick, leathery membrane forms over the area of damage. This membrane can be so large that it blocks the airway and causes suffocation, especially if the infection involves the larynx (voice box) and/or trachea (windpipe).

The toxin may also be absorbed into the body. It can then damage the heart, nerves and kidneys. Temporary paralysis can result from the effect of toxin on nerves.

Death from diphtheria occurs by either a membrane blocking the airway or toxin damaging the heart.

How Diphtheria Is Spread

Direct contact. Spread of diphtheria requires close, direct contact between people. For example, when an infected person coughs or sneezes, droplets containing bacteria may land in the nose or throat of another person. When diphtheria infects the skin, the disease can be spread if others come in contact with the sores.

Not airborne. In the past, outbreaks also occurred after people drank contaminated milk or ate contaminated milk products. Although diphtheria bacteria can survive outside the body for some hours, the disease is *not* spread through the air or from contaminated objects or dust.

Healthy carriers. Healthy people can be carriers of diphtheria bacteria; that is, the bacteria can live in the nose or throat of a person without causing any symptoms. Antibodies produced as a result of the vaccine protect the person from the disease by binding to the toxin so that it cannot damage cells. However, antibody against the toxin may not stop the bacteria from infecting the nose or throat.

So diphtheria germs can be spread by people who are not visibly sick. Persons ill with diphtheria are more likely than healthy carriers to spread the infection because they have larger quantities of bacteria in the throat.

Duration of contagious period. The risk of spreading the disease lasts as long as diphtheria bacteria remain in the nose or throat. Unless treated with appropriate antibiotics, most patients carry diphtheria bacteria for up to 4 weeks following illness. Diphtheria bacteria can be eradicated promptly with antibiotics, thereby making the patient non-contagious. The duration of carriage of diphtheria varies greatly in untreated patients; it may last weeks or months. Carriers remain contagious as long as the diphtheria bacteria are present.

The Illness

Symptoms. The time from exposure to diphtheria bacteria to becoming sick is usually 1 to 5 days. A sore throat, loss of appetite and low-grade fever are the first symptoms. Fever rarely is higher than 38.5°C (101.3°F). Within a day or two, pain in the throat becomes severe and the patient becomes increasingly ill, with marked weakness and decreased activity. The patient looks very sick.

Physical evidence. Grey-coloured patches of pus can be seen in the throat. The patches may combine to form a single membrane, which might cover the back of the throat, tonsils and soft palate. The grey membrane adheres to the surface and cannot be easily removed. The lymph glands in the neck become very swollen and tender. The entire neck may become swollen.

Recovery. Without treatment, the membrane begins to soften and break off in pieces after about a week, and symptoms of the illness gradually disappear.

Complications

Diphtheria is a severe disease. About 1 person in 10 (10%) with diphtheria still dies in spite of treatment.

Suffocation. Generally, the more severe the damage in the throat, the greater the chance of complications. In 1 out of 4 cases, the membrane extends down into the larynx and/or trachea. This form of diphtheria occurs most often in children under the age of 4. Signs of diphtheria affecting the larynx include hoarseness, noisy breathing (stridor) and increasingly difficult breathing. The membrane may get so big that it completely blocks the larynx, causing death by suffocation.

Heart failure. Another serious complication of diphtheria involves the heart. If enough toxin is absorbed into the body, it can damage the heart muscle. Heart failure and disturbance of heartbeat may occur, which may lead to death.

Nerve damage. Damage to nerves occurs in about 20% of cases. Nerves that lead to muscles are more often damaged than nerves carrying pain and other sensations. Paralysis develops 2 to 8 weeks after onset of the illness. Most patients recover from paralysis caused by diphtheria toxin, but recovery may be very slow.

Kidney failure. Diphtheria toxin can also damage blood vessels in the kidneys, leading to kidney failure.

Diagnosis

The diagnosis of diphtheria is based on the results of throat and nose swab cultures.

Treatment

Antitoxin. Whenever diphtheria is suspected, treatment should be started immediately, without waiting for test results. Swabs should be obtained for culture to confirm the diagnosis. Treatment of diphtheria consists of intravenous injection of antitoxin (this is different from the vaccine; see Text Box below for an explanation). Diphtheria antitoxin contains antibodies that neutralize or block the effects of the toxin.

> **Diphtheria antitoxin** is made by immunizing horses with diphtheria toxin and toxoid. (Toxoid is toxin that has been inactivated by chemical treatment so that it no longer is harmful, but still stimulates an immune response.) Horses are used because their size permits large amounts of serum to be prepared. The extracted serum is partially purified to concentrate the antibodies and to remove as many of the other proteins from the serum as possible (such as albumin).

Benefits of early treatment. The major benefit of treatment with antitoxin is prevention of damage to the heart. The sooner antitoxin treatment is started, the greater the benefit. If treatment begins within 48 hours of the start of illness, the death rate is about 5%. If treatment does not begin until the seventh day of illness, the death rate is 15–20%. Early treatment also reduces the risk of paralysis later on.

Antibiotics shorten contagious period. Antibiotics such as penicillin or erythromycin are very effective in eliminating diphtheria bacteria from the throat. Patients with diphtheria are treated with antibiotics to shorten the period of contagiousness. Antibiotic treatment, however, does not affect the duration or severity of the illness. The toxin that causes the disease has already been produced and absorbed by the body by the time treatment has begun.

Post-recovery. Persons who recover from diphtheria do not always develop immunity to the toxin. Diphtheria toxin is so potent that the amounts that cause disease may be too small to actually stimulate the immune system. Patients should therefore be fully immunized after recovery.

The Vaccine

Type of Vaccine

Inactivated bacterial toxin. The vaccine against diphtheria, known as diphtheria toxoid, was developed in 1923. It was discovered that combining diphtheria toxin with small amounts of formalin (a formaldehyde solution) made the toxin harmless, without affecting its ability to induce antibody. The vaccine, then, contains inactivated (harmless) diphtheria toxin.

It is now known that diphtheria toxin is composed of two subunits, A and B. Subunit B is required for attachment to and entry into cells; subunit A, which is the toxic portion, then causes the damage. Both antibody and antitoxin neutralize diphtheria toxin by combining with subunit B, preventing entry of the toxin into cells.

How Diphtheria Toxoid Is Made

Process. Diphtheria bacteria are grown in liquid culture. During growth, the bacteria release toxin into the liquid. After growth has occurred, the bacteria are removed. Formalin (a formaldehyde solution) is then added to inactivate the toxin and convert it to a toxoid. The final vaccine contains less than 0.02% (less than 200 parts per million) of residual formaldehyde. The product is further purified and concentrated to the required potency. The toxoid is then combined with alum (an aluminum salt), which enhances the immune response to the vaccine (i.e., it increases the amount of antibody produced).

Possible additive. A preservative called phenoxyethanol may be added, depending on which other vaccines are combined with the diphtheria toxoid. The vaccine does *not* contain thimerosal, a mercury-containing preservative.

Testing. Tests for potency (effectiveness), toxicity and sterility are carried out on all batches of vaccine, by both the manufacturer and the Bureau of Biologics and Radiopharmaceuticals. [See Chapter 2 for more detail.]

Available Forms of Diphtheria Toxoid

Combinations for infants and young children. Diphtheria toxoid is available in Canada either separately or combined with one or more other vaccines, including tetanus toxoid, acellular pertussis vaccine and inactivated polio vaccine.

The most commonly used combination in Canada is diphtheria toxoid, tetanus toxoid, acellular pertussis vaccine and inactivated polio vaccine (DTaP/IPV). The DTaP/IPV (a liquid) is used to dissolve the *Haemophilus influenzae* type b (Hib) vaccine (a powder). The combined product permits all five recommended vaccines for infants and young children to be given as a single injection.

Vaccines for older children and adults. Vaccines for children aged 7 and over and adults contain a lower amount of diphtheria toxoid than vaccines for young children (2 units per dose rather than 12–25 units). The reduced dose minimizes local reactions (e.g., swelling, redness) in older children and adults who have received their initial set of diphtheria vaccinations.

The *lower-dose formulation* is used in anyone aged 7 and over, whether it is an initial immunization or a booster (to enhance prior vaccination). There is no distinction made between these two circumstances for the following reason: it is impractical to manufacture and distribute a different vaccine to accommodate the extremely small number of people who would require the higher-dose formulation (i.e., those who can say, with absolute certainty, that they have never received the initial set of diphtheria vaccinations).

Diphtheria toxoid for older children and adults is available combined with tetanus toxoid (Td). (The lowercase "d" relates to the lower-dose formulation of diphtheria toxoid.) Lower-dose diphtheria toxoid is also available with tetanus toxoid and inactivated polio vaccine (Td/IPV), and with tetanus toxoid and the adult form [see Chapter 5, under *Available forms of pertussis vaccine*] of acellular pertussis vaccine (dTap).

How the Vaccine Is Given

Diphtheria toxoid (both adult and child formulations), whether alone or in combination with other vaccines, is supplied in a volume of 0.5 ml (one-tenth of a teaspoon).

Into muscle. Vaccines are administered by injection into muscle. In infants (children less than 12 months old), the vaccine is usually injected into the thigh because the muscle there is relatively large. In older children, the vaccine is usually given in the muscle of the upper arm.

It is important that diphtheria vaccines are injected into the muscle rather than into the overlying tissue beneath the skin (subcutaneous tissue). Injection into muscle with DTaP/IPV+Hib and other similar combination vaccines causes much milder local reaction than injection under the skin.

Schedule of Vaccination

Infants and children (under age 7). For routine immunization of young children in Canada, 4 doses of the combined DTaP/IPV+Hib vaccines are given: at 2, 4, 6 and 18 months. A booster dose of DTaP/IPV without Hib vaccine is given at 4 to 6 years of age. If a dose is missed or delayed for any reason, the series does not have to be started again.

Children (age 7 and over) and adults. For this group, whether as an initial vaccine or as a booster, a combination of tetanus toxoid and lower-dose diphtheria toxoid (Td) is recommended.

Boosters (to enhance prior vaccinations). A booster with either Td or dTap is recommended for teens (14 to 16 years of age) as a follow-up to the series they received as young children. A Td booster every 10 years is recommended for adults.

Duration of protection. Diphtheria toxoid does not provide lifelong immunity; therefore, boosters are recommended every 10 years.

Possible Side Effects of Diphtheria Toxoid

Diphtheria toxoid is one of the safest vaccines in current use. The most common reactions caused by diphtheria toxoid are redness, swelling, pain and tenderness at the site of the injection. The pain may cause babies to cry and be irritable. Local reactions are much more common in children and adults receiving boosters of the diphtheria toxoid than in infants receiving the first 3 doses. [For details of possible reactions after receiving the combined DTaP/IPV+Hib vaccine, see Chapter 5, Table 5.3.]

Reasons to Avoid or Delay Diphtheria Toxoid

Do not give. The National Advisory Committee on Immunization recognizes only one absolute contraindication to (a reason not to give) diphtheria vaccine: an anaphylactic reaction to a previous dose of the vaccine. Anaphylaxis is a severe allergic reaction involving one or more of the following: swelling of face or lips, difficulty breathing or shock (fall in blood pressure).

Do not delay. Vaccination should not be deferred or delayed because of minor illnesses, such as the common cold, with or without fever. Such infections do not increase the risk of side effects and do not interfere with the immune response to vaccination.

Delay. Moderate to severe illness, with or without fever, is a reason to delay routine immunization. This precaution should be taken to avoid adding any side effects of the vaccine on top of the effects of the illness itself.

The Results of Vaccination

Diphtheria toxoid prevents disease in most children and adults who have received all of the recommended doses. Those who do get diphtheria in spite of being fully vaccinated have a milder illness with fewer complications.

Even when most children are vaccinated, the bacteria do not disappear from the population. The vaccine prevents *disease* caused by diphtheria toxin, but does not prevent the persistence of diphtheria *bacteria* in the population.

Evidence that diphtheria toxoid works includes:
- the virtual disappearance of diphtheria cases in all countries in which immunization of infants and children is routine;
- the occurrence of recent epidemics of diphtheria (between 1990 and 1995) in Russia, the Ukraine and other countries of the former Soviet Union after marked falls in immunization rates followed by control of the outbreaks with mass immunization;
- an 85–90% reduction in the number of cases in fully immunized children during outbreaks of diphtheria;
- milder disease and fewer complications in fully immunized persons.

Outbreaks in other countries. Indirect evidence supporting the effectiveness of diphtheria toxoid is provided by the recent experience in Russia, the Ukraine and other states of the former Soviet Union. Following an anti-vaccination campaign, which was fuelled by many stories appearing on TV and in newspapers about the alleged dangers of vaccines, a marked decrease in the number of children being vaccinated occurred in the late 1980s.

The decline in vaccination was quickly followed by a very large diphtheria epidemic: between 1990 and 1995, over 100,000 cases of diphtheria and more than 1,200 disease-related deaths occurred in the Ukraine and Russia alone. The epidemic was eventually controlled by a mass vaccination program.

Summary

- Immunization with diphtheria toxoid has been extremely effective in preventing diphtheria.
- In Canada and the United States, most parents and doctors today have not seen a child with diphtheria. The success of routine vaccination is confirmed by the fact that fewer than 5 cases per year have been reported in Canada since 1983.
- However, it is very important not to be fooled. Diphtheria bacteria have not disappeared, and the disease will return if routine vaccination is discontinued. This fact is evidenced by the recent occurrences in the Ukraine and Russia.
- The vaccine is very safe. Although local adverse reactions do occur, serious or life-threatening events caused by diphtheria toxoid are extremely rare, if they occur at all.

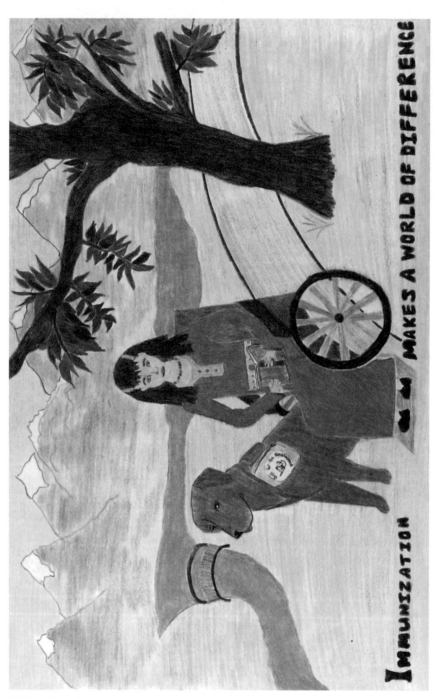

Kaitlyn La Rose, Saskatoon, Saskatchewan

CHAPTER 4

Tetanus

Tetanus is a disease caused by a toxin (poison). The toxin is made by bacteria called *Clostridium tetani*. The toxin blocks normal control of nerve reflexes in the spinal cord. As a result, intense stimulation of muscles occurs throughout the body. These muscle contractions last a long time and are very painful. They may cause death by interfering with breathing. The disease is sometimes called lockjaw because the jaws may become very tightly clenched with spasms of the jaw muscles.

Tetanus bacteria have the ability to form spores. Spores are a special form of the bacteria that have an external coating. This coating protects the bacteria in the environment. Tetanus spores can survive for many years outside the body and are very widespread in our environment. They live not only in dirt, but also in dust — even in dust within hospitals! Anyone who lacks antibody to tetanus is susceptible to the disease.

The "T" in the combination DTaP vaccine stands for tetanus.

A History of Tetanus

Before Vaccine

The bacteria that cause tetanus were identified in 1890. In 1891, it was discovered that a toxin (poison) made by tetanus bacteria caused the illness.

Before tetanus vaccination became routine in the 1940s, 60 to 75 cases of tetanus occurred every year in Canada, with 40 to 50 deaths. Tetanus has always been more common in males than in females: most cases of tetanus occurred in newborns, but it also affected older boys and young men. Before the vaccine was available, tetanus killed many wounded soldiers during every war.

The introduction of tetanus antitoxin (this is different from the vaccine; see box for explanation) neutralized the effect of tetanus toxin and improved the care of wounds. This led to a decline in the number of cases and deaths after 1920 in Canada, the United States and other industrialized countries. However, tetanus remained a major killer in most other parts of the world.

Even until 1984, newborn babies were getting the disease through infection of the stump of the umbilical cord. That year, more than 1 million newborn babies died of tetanus throughout the world. In countries that do not vaccinate against tetanus, this disease still kills.

Tetanus antitoxin is made by immunizing horses with tetanus toxin and toxoid. (Toxoid is toxin that has been inactivated by chemical treatment so that it no longer is harmful, but still stimulates an immune response.) Horses are used because their size permits large amounts of serum to be prepared. The extracted serum is partially purified to concentrate the antibodies and to remove as many of the other proteins in the serum as possible (such as albumin).

After Vaccine

Isolation and purification of tetanus toxin led to the development of tetanus toxoid (the vaccine against tetanus). The toxoid became available in Canada and the United States in 1938. Routine use of tetanus toxoid during World War II had a dramatic effect: the rate of tetanus among wounded soldiers in American and British forces was over 30 times less frequent than it had been in World War I.

The success of tetanus toxoid in preventing tetanus in soldiers during World War II led to the recommendation, in 1944, of routine immunization of all children in Canada and the United States. It was advised for the following reasons:
- the universal presence of tetanus spores in the environment;
- the high death rate from tetanus (10–20%) even with treatment;
- the safety and effectiveness of the vaccine.

The frequency of tetanus has declined in all countries that have programs to vaccinate all infants. During the past 15 years, there have been fewer than 2 cases per year in Canada.

The Germ

Tetanus germs exist in two forms: growing bacteria and spores. Tetanus bacteria live in the large bowel of humans and many animals, including horses, dogs, guinea pigs, sheep and cattle. The tetanus germ is strictly anaerobic, which means that it can grow and multiply only in the absence of oxygen.

The bacteria produce spores as they grow in the intestines. The spores are excreted in the feces, contaminating the environment in which the person or animal lives.

Tetanus spores are actually tough survival pods. They are covered with a special coating that allows them to survive outside the body. The spores do not multiply, but are able to stay alive in soil and dust (even in dust within hospitals!) for many years. Therefore, the bacteria can never be eradicated. They cannot be killed by boiling or by most disinfectants.

How It Causes Illness

The disease begins when spores present in dirt or dust make their way to the tissue below the skin via an injury such as a puncture, laceration or bite. The severity of the injury does not matter — tetanus can occur even after very minor injuries that do not require medical attention, such as cuts, scrapes and bites. Puncture wounds, such as those that occur by stepping on a nail, have an increased risk of tetanus compared with cuts because of the difficulty of thoroughly cleaning a wound of that nature.

Once inside the tissue, the spores can change into bacteria only if the amount of oxygen in the wound is very low. (Low oxygen conditions may occur if the wound is not cleaned properly and damaged or dead tissue is not removed.) As the bacteria grow and die, they release toxin into the tissue.

Tetanus toxin is a nerve poison, and it is one of the most powerful poisons in nature. The smallest dose that will kill an adult is less than 2 ng (2 nanograms is less than 2 billionth of a gram, or 0.000000002 g). The toxin is released by tetanus bacteria and reaches the spinal cord through the bloodstream and by travelling up nerves from the muscle.

The toxin blocks the activity of nerve cells in the spinal cord and brain so that normal control of spinal reflexes is lost. This loss of control of spinal reflexes leads to excess stimulation of muscles throughout the body. As a result, muscles contract uncontrollably, causing severe pain.

How Tetanus Is Spread

Poisonous spores. Tetanus is unique among all of the infections prevented by vaccines in that it is not contagious: it does not spread from person to person. Infection is acquired by exposure to spores in the environment. In order to cause disease, the spores must be introduced through the skin as a result of an injury such as a puncture, laceration or bite. Only if the proper conditions of low oxygen are present can the spores begin to grow and release toxin.

Anyone who lacks antibody to tetanus is susceptible to the disease.

Contaminated soil and dust. The most common source of exposure to tetanus spores is soil. Studies have shown that almost one-third of soil samples collected in North America contain tetanus spores. Spores have also been found in street dust as well as in dust in houses and hospitals.

The Illness

Symptoms. Most cases of tetanus begin within 1 to 7 days of injury. Rarely, symptoms have been delayed for up to 60 days after injury.

Physical evidence. The hallmark of tetanus is muscle spasm: prolonged, uncontrollable contraction of muscle. The spasms are very painful. They may be triggered by mild stimuli, such as sudden noise or movement. The first symptom is usually spasm of the jaw muscles, which explains the common name for the disease, "lockjaw." Swallowing may become very difficult. This is followed by spasms of muscles in the face, neck, chest, abdomen, arms and legs.

All muscles involved may go into spasm at the same time. The patient remains alert and aware of surroundings in spite of repeated spasms. The spasms remain frequent and intense for 1 to 4 weeks and then gradually subside.

Complications

Tetanus is a severe disease. Even with treatment in a modern intensive care unit, the death rate is 10–20%. Death is much more frequent in the many parts of the world that lack modern facilities, especially for newborn infants who get tetanus as a result of contamination of the umbilical cord or stump shortly after birth.

Suffocation. A spasm of the muscles of the vocal cords can result in immediate death by blocking the airway.

Other complications of tetanus include:
- choking spells because of difficulty swallowing;
- weight loss because of poor eating;
- bone fractures from severe muscle spasms;
- problems associated with any severe prolonged illness requiring intensive care, such as pneumonia (infection of the lungs) and skin ulcers;
- lasting difficulties with speech, memory and mental function.

Diagnosis

The diagnosis of tetanus is based on the findings of typical muscle spasms developing within days of an injury. Cultures of infected wounds are usually not helpful because of the difficulty of finding tetanus bacteria among the many other bacteria present in pus.

Treatment

Treatment of tetanus involves:
- surgical cleaning of the wound and removal of any dead tissue containing tetanus spores;
- killing tetanus bacteria in the wound with antibiotics to prevent production of more toxin;
- neutralizing "free floating" toxin in the wound and blood with tetanus immune globulin [see next paragraph] to prevent toxin from binding to nerve cells;
- relieving and preventing muscle spasms with drugs.

Tetanus immune globulin, or TIG, is derived from blood donated by adult volunteers. The volunteers have been repeatedly vaccinated with tetanus toxoid vaccine so that they develop high concentrations of antibodies to tetanus toxin. Plasma (the liquid part of the blood) is obtained from the blood samples of these volunteers and the antibodies are purified to produce TIG.

TIG is given by injection into a muscle. Volunteers are tested to be certain that they are not infected with HIV, hepatitis B, hepatitis C or other blood-borne viruses. No infections with these viruses have occurred as the result of use of TIG.

Post-recovery. So little toxin is released during the course of the disease that survivors usually do not become immune to tetanus. There have been recurrent cases; so, all survivors should be fully immunized for future protection.

The Vaccine

Type of Vaccine

Inactivated bacterial toxin. The vaccine against tetanus, known as tetanus toxoid, consists of inactivated tetanus toxin. To make the toxin inactive, it is treated with formalin (a formaldehyde solution). Although this treatment inactivates the ability of the toxin to make someone sick, it doesn't affect its ability to induce an immune response when injected into the body. The antibodies induced by the tetanus toxoid are able to neutralize the toxin and prevent binding of toxin to nerve cells.

How Tetanus Toxoid Is Made

Process. Tetanus bacteria are grown in liquid culture, into which they release toxin. The fluid is filtered to remove the bacteria. The toxin is then purified from the fluid, concentrated to the required potency, and treated with formaldehyde to make it a harmless toxoid. The final vaccine contains less than 0.02% (less than 200 parts per million) of formaldehyde. The toxoid is combined with alum (an aluminum salt), which enhances the immune response to the vaccine.

Possible additive. Phenoxyethanol is added as a preservative if required, depending on which other vaccines are combined with tetanus toxoid. The vaccine does *not* contain thimerosal, a mercury-containing preservative.

Testing. Mandatory tests for potency (effectiveness), toxicity and sterility are carried out on all lots (batches) of vaccine before they are allowed to be distributed [see Chapter 2, under *Vaccine safety*].

Available Forms of Tetanus Toxoid

Combinations for infants and children. Tetanus toxoid is available in Canada either separately or combined with one or more vaccines, including diphtheria toxoid, acellular pertussis vaccine and inactivated polio vaccine. Unless there is known allergy to diphtheria toxoid, it is recommended that tetanus toxoid always be given in combination with diphtheria toxoid.

The most commonly used combination in Canada is diphtheria toxoid, tetanus toxoid, acellular pertussis vaccine and inactivated polio vaccine (DTaP/IPV). The DTaP/IPV (a liquid) is used to dissolve the *Haemophilus influenzae* type b (Hib) vaccine (a powder). The combined product permits all five recommended vaccines for infants and young children to be given as a single injection.

Vaccines for older children and adults. Tetanus toxoid for older children (age 7 and over) and adults is available combined with diphtheria toxoid (Td). (The lowercase "d" relates to the lower-dose formulation of diphtheria toxoid used in anyone aged 7 and over, whether it is an initial immunization or a booster.) [See Chapter 3, under *Available forms of diphtheria toxoid*, for the reason no distinction is made between the two circumstances.] Tetanus toxoid is also available with lower-dose diphtheria toxoid and inactivated polio vaccine (Td/IPV), and with lower-dose diphtheria toxoid and the adult form of acellular pertussis vaccine (dTap). [For more information about the adult form of pertussis vaccine, see Chapter 5, under *Available forms of pertussis vaccine*.]

How the Vaccine Is Given

Tetanus toxoid, whether alone or in combination with other vaccines, is supplied in a volume of 0.5 ml (one-tenth of a teaspoon).

Into muscle. The vaccine is administered by injection into muscle. In infants (less than 12 months), the vaccine is usually injected into the thigh because the muscle there is relatively large. In older children, the vaccine is usually given in the muscle of the upper arm.

It is important that tetanus toxoid is injected into muscle rather than into the tissue beneath the skin (subcutaneous tissue). Injection into muscle with vaccines that contain alum (tetanus, diphtheria and combinations of tetanus and diphtheria with pertussis, IPV and Hib) causes much milder local reaction (e.g., redness, swelling) than injection under the skin.

Schedule of Vaccination

Infants and children (under age 7). For routine immunization of young children in Canada, 4 doses of the combined DTaP/IPV+Hib vaccine are given: at 2, 4, 6 and 18 months. A booster dose of DTaP/IPV without Hib vaccine is given at 4 to 6 years of age. If a dose is missed or delayed for any reason, the series does not have to be started again.

Children (age 7 and over) and adults. For this group, whether as an initial vaccine or as a booster, a combination of tetanus toxoid and lower-dose diphtheria toxoid (Td) is recommended.

Boosters (to enhance prior vaccinations). Boosters of Td (tetanus and lower-dose diphtheria) and dTap (tetanus, lower-dose diphtheria and the adult form of acellular pertussis vaccine) are available for teens (14 to 16 years of age) as a follow-up to the series they received as young children. A Td booster every 10 years is recommended for adults.

Duration of protection. Tetanus toxoid does not provide lifelong immunity. Boosters every 10 years are therefore recommended [see above].

Possible Side Effects of Tetanus Toxoid

Local reactions. Redness, swelling, pain and tenderness at the site of injection are the most common reactions occurring after injection of tetanus toxoid. [For details of possible reactions after receiving the combined DTaP/IPV + Hib vaccine, see Chapter 5, Table 5.3.] The likelihood of local reactions increases with the number of doses given. Most people have local reactions after boosters. The severity of local reactions from boosters is related to the concentration of tetanus antitoxin present in the body at the time of injection.

Severe local reactions (extensive swelling, redness and pain) occur in less than 2% of those given boosters. Most severe local reactions occur in persons who have received boosters too often (i.e., more than once every 10 years). Although the pain and tenderness may be severe enough to limit mobility of the arm for a few days, the reactions cause no permanent damage.

Other mild reactions following tetanus vaccination include swollen lymph glands (especially those near the site of injection), fever, headache and muscle aches.

Allergic reactions (usually hives) do occur, but are rare. Serious allergic reactions were reported in 1 out of 100,000 United States Air Force recruits given tetanus toxoid boosters. As tetanus toxoid is usually given in combination with other vaccines, the cause of a reaction may not be easy to identify. Severe allergic reactions are much less common in infants and young children than in adults. They can be fatal if not treated promptly.

Adverse neurologic events have been reported following administration of tetanus toxoid. It has not been possible to prove whether such reactions have been merely coincidental or whether the vaccine has actually caused the reactions.

The most common neurologic events reported have been paralysis and changes in sensation resulting from damage to peripheral nerves. In the cases involving nerve damage, the pattern of involvement of the affected nerves is similar to that seen in serum sickness, or a severe allergic reaction that can be caused by many different drugs. The frequency of adverse neurologic events following vaccination is estimated to be less than 1 per million doses of vaccine.

Reasons to Avoid or Delay Tetanus Toxoid

Do not give. The National Advisory Committee on Immunization recognizes only one absolute reason not to give tetanus vaccine: an anaphylactic reaction to a previous dose of the vaccine. Anaphylaxis is a severe allergic reaction involving one or more of the following: swelling of face or lips, difficulty breathing or shock (fall in blood pressure).

Do not delay. Vaccination should not be deferred or delayed because of minor illnesses, such as the common cold, with or without fever. Such infections do not increase the risk of side effects and do not interfere with the immune response to vaccination.

Delay. Moderate to severe illness, with or without fever, is a reason to delay routine immunization. This precaution should be taken to avoid the possibility of adding any side effects of the vaccine on top of the effects of the illness itself.

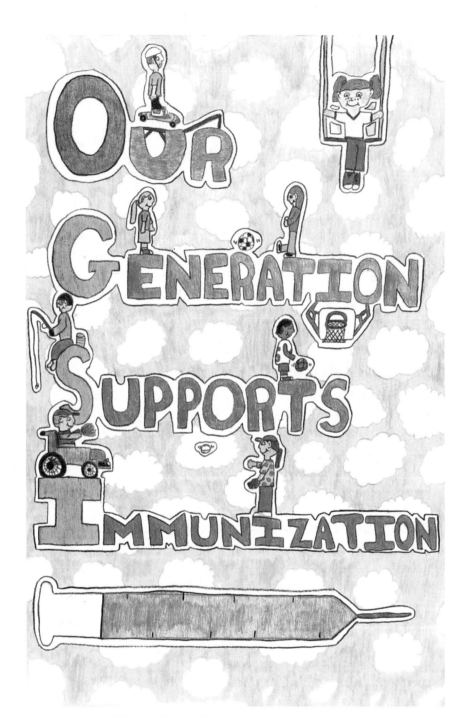

Samantha Lawrence, Bridgewater, Nova Scotia

The Results of Vaccination

Tetanus is extremely rare in anyone who is up-to-date with recommended tetanus immunization. In Canada and the United States today, most cases of tetanus occur in persons over age 60 who either have never had the vaccine or have not had a booster for more than 10 years. The only cases of tetanus in children in the U.S. over the past 20 years have been in those who were not immunized because their parents did not believe in immunization.

It is clear from experience with mass immunization of soldiers as well as with mass programs to prevent tetanus in newborns in underdeveloped countries that tetanus toxoid is highly effective.

Evidence that tetanus toxoid works includes:
- the virtual disappearance of tetanus cases in all countries in which immunization of infants and children is routine;
- the extreme rarity of tetanus in fully immunized persons;
- controlled studies showing marked decline in tetanus in newborn infants following immunization of mothers during pregnancy;
- the rarity of tetanus in Canadian, American and British soldiers in World War II following implementation of vaccination of all recruits.

Summary

- Tetanus toxoid is one of the safest and most effective vaccines.
- Tetanus is not contagious: it does not spread from person to person. Infection is acquired by exposure to spores in the environment.
- Because tetanus spores occur everywhere in our environment, the only effective means of preventing tetanus is vaccination.

- The vaccine prevents *disease* caused by the toxin. Vaccination cannot eradicate or diminish the presence of tetanus spores in the environment.
- In countries that do not vaccinate against tetanus, this disease still kills.
- Following the vaccine series in infancy and early childhood, booster doses every 10 years are recommended to ensure long-term protection against tetanus.

CHAPTER 5

Pertussis

Pertussis is a respiratory infection caused by bacteria called *Bordetella pertussis*. Pertussis is also known as "whooping cough" because the major symptom is severe spells of coughing followed by a whoop sound before the next breath. The illness lasts many weeks.

The "aP" in the combination DTaP vaccine stands for acellular pertussis. The acellular vaccine is the most current type of pertussis vaccine used in Canada. It replaced the whole cell pertussis vaccine (used in the former DPT combination) in 1997.

A History of Pertussis

Before Vaccine

Pertussis used to kill many children. In the early 1900s, 5 out of every 1,000 children born in the United States and Canada died of pertussis before they reached their fifth birthday. Prior to routine vaccination against pertussis, there were between 30,000 and 50,000 cases every year in Canada with 50 to 100 deaths. Most deaths involved infants (babies less than 12 months old).

Fortunately, the death rate from pertussis declined in developed countries long before vaccine or antibiotics became available. For example, in Canada, the United States and England, infant deaths from pertussis decreased by over 70% between 1900 and 1940. Factors that contributed to this decrease included better nutrition, less overcrowding and smaller families.

These changes reduced the risk of exposure of young infants to pertussis, but almost 100% of children had the infection by 10 to 12 years of age. Although there were fewer pertussis *deaths*, there was still no decrease in the number of pertussis *cases* until the vaccine became available.

After Vaccine

Widespread use of pertussis vaccine has led to an even more rapid decline in the death rate than that experienced in the pre-vaccine era. Now, pertussis kills between 1 and 3 infants every year in Canada. There has also been a marked drop in the number of cases of pertussis, but several thousand cases and several pertussis-related deaths still occur every year in Canada. Outbreaks of pertussis happen every 3 to 5 years in Canada. Almost two-thirds of cases occur between July and December, peaking between August and October.

Studies in Nova Scotia provide the best estimate of the frequency of pertussis cases in Canada today. Intense efforts were made to record all cases between 1986 and 1988; the results show that the average rate of pertussis each year was 74 for every 100,000 people. During an epidemic in this period, the rate was five times higher than the lowest recorded rate. Three-quarters of the cases occurred in children under the age of 5.

The rate of pertussis is 10 times lower in Nova Scotia (where most children are vaccinated) than in Sweden (where pertussis vaccine was not used between 1979 and the mid-1990s). Similarly, the rate of pertussis is much higher in Italy than in Canada because pertussis vaccine has not been used regularly there until recently. By 5 years of age, 25% of children in Italy have had pertussis. Following the introduction of routine vaccination with pertussis vaccine in Sweden and Italy, the rate of pertussis declined markedly in both countries.

The Germ

Bordetella pertussis bacteria were first identified in 1906. Over the past 15 years, a number of proteins of the cell wall of the bacteria have been identified, which both damage the body and stimulate immune responses.

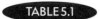

TABLE 5.1

The role of components of pertussis bacteria in producing disease and immunity, by level of importance

COMPONENTS OF PERTUSSIS BACTERIA	ROLE IN PRODUCING DISEASE		ROLE IN PRODUCING IMMUNITY
	Attachment to cells	Damage to cells	
Pertussis toxin (PT)	2	2	2
Filamentous hemagglutinin (FHA)	2	0	0
Pertactin (PER)	1	1	2
Fimbria 2 (FIM 2)	2	0	2
Fimbria 3 (FIM 3)	2	0	2
Adenylate cyclase	0	2	?

Scale: 2 = Important 1 = Possibly important 0 = Not important ? = Importance unknown

How It Causes Illness

Pertussis is unusual compared with other infections in that the bacteria remain on the surface of the airways and do not invade the tissues. After exposure to an infected person, the next stage of infection [see Table 5.2] is attachment of the bacteria to cells that line the nose, throat and bronchi (the air tubes in the lungs). Pertussis toxin, filamentous hemagglutinin, fimbriae and pertactin, which are proteins on the outer surface of the bacteria, are all involved in binding pertussis bacteria to cells lining the airways.

Pertussis toxin, adenylate cyclase and other toxins damage the cells, especially cells with small hair-like projections called cilia. The cilia normally move continuously in waves; this is how mucus is carried up from the lungs and the bronchi into the mouth, where it is swallowed. This process is important because as the mucus travels, it coats the surface of the nose, throat and airways of the lungs, forming a protective layer. Damage to the cilia interferes with the normal transfer of mucus from the airways to the mouth. In addition, excess mucus is made because of the inflammation.

The combination of damage to cells, excess mucus, and failure to move the mucus out of the airways leads to the attacks of coughing typical of pertussis.

TABLE 5.2

Factors involved in the stages of pertussis infection

STAGE OF INFECTION	FACTORS INVOLVED
Exposure to pertussis bacteria	Close contact with someone infected with pertussis bacteria
Attachment of bacteria to cells	PT, FHA, FIM, PER
Damage to cells Impairment of movement of mucus Runny nose Paroxysmal (with spasms) cough	PT, adenylate cyclase, other toxins
Recovery	Immune system responds to infection by producing antibody

Pertussis toxin and adenylate cyclase also interfere with the normal function of white blood cells, which defend the body against infection.

The immune system responds to infection with pertussis bacteria by making antibody against pertussis toxin, filamentous hemagglutinin, fimbriae 2 and 3, pertactin, and other components of the bacteria [see Table 5.1 above].

How Pertussis Is Spread

Direct contact. Spread of pertussis requires close, direct contact between people. An infected person may cough or sneeze, spreading droplets containing many pertussis bacteria. These droplets may land in the nose or throat of another person. Indirect spread through the air or on contaminated toys or other objects occurs very rarely, if at all.

Very contagious. In a home environment where close contact of individuals is frequent, it is estimated that 9 out of 10 susceptible persons (i.e., those with no immunity to the disease) will get pertussis. Spread of infection is somewhat less frequent in school settings because contact between children there is not as frequent or as close as it is in the home.

Duration of contagious period. Pertussis is most contagious during the first 2 weeks, when symptoms resemble those of a common cold. Contagiousness declines rapidly after that, but may last up to 3 weeks. Patients are no longer contagious after 5 days of treatment with antibiotics.

The Illness

Symptoms in children. In most cases, symptoms first occur 7 to 10 days after exposure to the bacteria, but may be delayed for up to 20 days. Pertussis usually begins with a runny nose. Often, the discharge from the nose is profuse. Temperature is usually normal or only slightly increased. After a few days to a week, the child begins to cough.

Characteristic cough. The cough gets worse and worse until "spells" begin, during which the child coughs without being able to stop to take a breath. At the end of a coughing spell, the characteristic whoop sound may occur as the child takes a very deep breath.

Between coughing spells, the person often appears quite normal. However, young infants may become exhausted by frequent, severe coughing episodes. Because they often vomit after coughing and feed poorly when ill, infants may lose weight. Coughing may be triggered by many stimuli, including eating, drinking, crying and laughing.

Slow recovery. After 1 to 2 weeks of severe coughing spells, the child begins to get better. The spells gradually subside over an additional few weeks. The typical illness lasts 6 to 12 weeks. For several months after recovering from pertussis, children may experience coughing spells triggered by anything that irritates the airways, including a common cold, cigarette smoke or even cold air.

Infection in teens and adults. Adolescents and adults who are infected with pertussis often have an illness quite similar to that seen in infants and children. Almost all have some type of cough, which lasts more than 3 weeks in 80% of cases. Although whooping is rare in adolescents and adults, the cough occurs in prolonged paroxysms (spasms) in almost two-thirds of patients and disturbs sleep in half.

Complications

Minor complications of pertussis include nosebleeds and small hemorrhages in the white of the eye as a result of forceful coughing. Swelling of the face may also occur. Ear infections are very common.

Severe complications. In most children with pertussis, small areas of the lungs collapse because plugs of thick mucus block the airways. Frequently, such areas are invaded by other bacteria or viruses, causing pneumonia (an infection of the lungs).

About 20–30% of infants (babies less than 12 months old) with pertussis are so sick that they are admitted to hospital. Young infants may have spells when they stop breathing instead of coughing. Such attacks may lead to convulsions and coma. Brain damage occurs in approximately 1 out of every 400 infants who are hospitalized with pertussis. Pertussis can lead to brain damage in at least three ways:
• by interfering with blood supply to the brain during severe coughing spells;

- by causing the infant to stop breathing;
- by causing the blood vessels in the brain to rupture during coughing spells and bleed into the brain.

About 1 of every 400 infants hospitalized with pertussis dies as a result of either pneumonia or brain damage.

Learning and behaviour problems. Studies in Britain show that children who had pertussis in infancy have a much higher rate of learning and behaviour problems than children who did not have the infection.

In adolescents and adults. Complications of pertussis are much less frequent in adolescents and adults than in infants, but the illness is prolonged and frequently causes school absenteeism and lost workdays.

Diagnosis

Bacterial cultures. The diagnosis of pertussis can be confirmed by performing a culture for the bacteria on fluid from the nose. Cultures are positive most often in the first 2 weeks of illness. By the third week, less than half of the cultures are still positive. Cultures are often negative in those who have had pertussis vaccine and in those with mild illness.

New techniques have been developed that are better than performing a culture to confirm pertussis. These involve either measuring antibody responses in the blood or detecting DNA of pertussis bacteria in respiratory secretions. Such methods are widely available in Canada.

In adolescents and adults. Pertussis should be considered as a possible diagnosis in any adolescent or adult with a cough persisting more than 2 weeks.

Treatment

Antibiotics. Although a number of antibiotics can destroy pertussis bacteria, the results of antibiotic treatment of patients with pertussis have been disappointing. Erythromycin and similar antibiotics (not penicillin or amoxicillin) can get rid of pertussis bacteria from the nose and throat.

Early treatment. If treatment is started during the first 2 weeks of illness, coughing may not last as long as in patients who do not receive medication. However, antibiotics have very little effect on patients with coughing spasms; at that point, the illness is too advanced to respond to treatment.

Post-recovery. Subsequent attacks of full-blown pertussis are very rare. Pertussis can occur more than once, but symptoms are usually mild or absent in repeat infections. Recent research suggests that immunity following infection is not lifelong. Patients should therefore be fully immunized after recovery.

The Vaccine

Type of Vaccine

Purified bacterial proteins. The pertussis vaccine currently used in Canada (since 1997) is called *acellular pertussis vaccine*. It is not possible to get the disease from the vaccine because it contains purified proteins rather than dead, intact bacteria as in the original whole cell pertussis vaccine.

Researchers have identified the proteins in the pertussis bacteria that are responsible for inducing immunity to pertussis. With the development of methods to extract and purify these proteins, scientists have been able to produce the acellular pertussis vaccine. Recent studies of these new pertussis vaccines suggest that antibodies against pertussis toxin, fimbriae and pertactin may be the most important in protecting against infection and reducing the severity of disease [see Table 5.1 earlier in this Chapter].

How Pertussis Vaccine Is Made

History of acellular vaccine. The original acellular vaccines, first made in Japan in 1981, consisted of purified extracts of fluid in which pertussis bacteria had been grown. Six Japanese manufacturers produced acellular vaccines that varied markedly in composition. Since then, manufacturers in Canada, the United States and Europe have developed new methods to separate and purify the pertussis proteins.

The vaccines, made by several manufacturers, differ in both the number and concentration of the proteins in each dose. The vaccine developed and manufactured in Canada, however, is the only acellular pertussis vaccine to contain five purified proteins: pertussis toxin, filamentous hemagglutinin, pertactin, and fimbriae 2 and 3.

The acellular pertussis vaccine replaced the whole cell pertussis vaccine in 1997 in Canada. [See the previous section for the difference between the two vaccines.]

Process. The pertussis proteins are purified, sterilized and their concentrations adjusted to the desired level. The vaccine can then be combined with diphtheria and tetanus toxoids. In Canada, a 5-in-1 shot containing diphtheria and tetanus toxoids, acellular pertussis vaccine, inactivated polio vaccine and *Haemophilus influenzae* type b vaccine (DTaP/IPV+Hib vaccine) was licensed in 1997 and is used in all provinces and territories. More than 3 million doses of the combination vaccine have been given.

The final product contains less than 0.02% (less than 200 parts per million) of residual formaldehyde used in making the diphtheria and tetanus toxoids, and alum (an aluminum salt), which enhances the immune response to the vaccine.

Additive. Phenoxyethanol is added as a preservative to prevent bacterial contamination of the vaccine. The vaccine does *not* contain thimerosal, a mercury-containing preservative.

Testing. Mandatory tests for potency (effectiveness), toxicity and sterility are carried out on all lots (batches) of vaccine before they can be distributed [see Chapter 2].

Available Forms of Pertussis Vaccine

Combinations for infants and children. Acellular pertussis vaccine is most often used in a combination product that also contains diphtheria and tetanus toxoids (DTaP). In Canada, DTaP is combined with inactivated polio vaccine (IPV). This liquid combination is then used to dissolve the *Haemophilus influenzae* type b (Hib) vaccine (a powder) so that all five vaccines can be given to infants and young children as a single injection.

Vaccines for adolescents and adults. A special form of the acellular pertussis vaccine was developed specifically for older children and adults (ages 12 to 65). It is licensed in Canada as a combined vaccine containing tetanus toxoid, lower-dose diphtheria toxoid, and adult acellular pertussis vaccine (dTap). The special form contains a lower amount of pertussis toxoid and filamentous hemagglutinin than the infant vaccine, but is otherwise the same. It can be used as a booster or as an initial dose.

How the Vaccine Is Given

Into muscle. The acellular pertussis vaccine — alone or combined with diphtheria, polio, tetanus and Hib vaccines — is given by injection into muscle. In infants (children less than 12 months old), the vaccine is usually injected into the thigh because the muscle there is relatively large. In older children, the vaccine is usually given in the muscle of the upper arm.

It is important that pertussis vaccines are injected into muscle rather than into the tissue beneath the skin (subcutaneous tissue). Injection into muscle with vaccines that contain alum causes much milder local reaction (e.g., redness, swelling) than injection under the skin.

Schedule of Vaccination

Infants and children (under age 12). Three doses of DTaP are given (at 2, 4 and 6 months of age), followed by boosters at 18 months and

4 to 6 years of age. If a dose is missed or delayed for any reason, the series does not have to be started again.

Boosters (to enhance prior vaccinations) for ages 12 to 65. Reactions are much less common with the acellular vaccine than with the whole cell pertussis vaccine, which was used prior to 1997. It is therefore possible to give boosters to adolescents and adults. The new adult form of the acellular pertussis vaccine is safe and induces strong immune responses in people in this age range.

It is expected that a booster dose in adolescents and/or young adults will be very helpful in prolonging protection against pertussis. Boosters to adolescents should decrease school outbreaks and disease in this age group; boosters in general will reduce the spread of infection to unimmunized infants.

Duration of protection. It is not yet clear how long immunity lasts after vaccination with the acellular vaccine. Studies of infants in Sweden and Italy show that they were protected for more than 3 years following vaccination at 2, 4 and 6 months of age. There was no decrease in immunity over this period.

With the five-dose Canadian immunization schedule of acellular pertussis vaccine (at 2, 4, 6 and 18 months and at 4 to 6 years of age), protection should last throughout childhood. But, it is likely that immunity will decrease over time so that adolescents and young adults become susceptible. A booster dose has therefore been recommended for adolescents. At the time of writing, parents must pay for the booster vaccine in most provinces and territories.

Possible Side Effects of Pertussis Vaccine

Minor side effects of acellular pertussis vaccine usually start within 12 to 24 hours of vaccination. Symptoms that begin more than 48 hours after vaccination are most likely caused by something other than the vaccine. Side effects following the acellular vaccine are much less frequent and much less severe than those seen with the whole cell vaccine, which was used prior to 1997.

Generalized side effects in infants include fever, fussiness, crying, drowsiness, reduced appetite and vomiting. Such events are usually mild and occur in about half of vaccinated infants.

Localized side effects (redness, swelling, pain and tenderness at the site of injection) occur singly or in combination in about 1 out of 4 children. A few children develop firm lumps at the site of injection, which may not appear for days or weeks. These lumps are the result of a scar forming at the site of inflammation caused by the vaccine. They almost always disappear with time. Very rarely, an abscess forms at the site of injection and usually heals without treatment.

Generalized and localized side effects are rarely severe: high fever equal to or greater than 40°C (104°F) occurs after fewer than 1 in 3,000 doses; prolonged crying after fewer than 1 in 300; and severe fussiness after fewer than 1 in 100. [See below for details on side effects.]

Table 5.3 below summarizes results from Canadian studies in which more than 1,000 infants received a total of 3,272 doses of acellular pertussis vaccine as part of the combined DTaP/IPV+Hib vaccine.

TABLE 5.3

Severity and frequency of side effects reported in more than 1,000 Canadian infants given doses of DTaP/IPV+Hib vaccine (3,272 in all) at 2, 4 and 6 months of age*

SIDE EFFECT	SEVERITY	FREQUENCY
Fever	Greater than 38°C (100.4°F)	1 in 6 (16.7%)
	Greater than 40°C (104°F)	1 in 3,000 (0.03%)
Fussiness	Any	1 in 2 (45.2%)
	Severe	1 in 100 (1.3%)
Crying	Any	1 in 3 (30.2%)
	Longer than 3 hours	1 in 333 (0.3%)
Local redness	Any	1 in 9 (11.5%)
	Greater than 30 mm (1.3 in.) wide	1 in 40 (2.5%)
Local tenderness or pain	Any	1 in 5 (22.3%)
	Severe	1 in 34 (2.9%)

* Results are per dose, not per child.

Research into localized side effects. Areas of local redness and swelling after vaccines containing acellular pertussis vaccine are usually larger after the fourth and fifth doses (the boosters given at 18 months and ages 4 to 6) than after the first 3 injections.

A study was done of 52 Canadian children who had received 4 doses of acellular pertussis (as DTaP/IPV+Hib vaccine) at 2, 4, 6 and 18 months of age. After the fifth dose of acellular pertussis at 4 to 6 years of age, half of the children had redness and swelling greater than 5 cm (2 in.) of the upper arm. However, only 2% (1 child) had moderate to severe pain and none of the children had limitation of movement of their arm because of pain or tenderness.

Research is underway to determine the causes of the large local reactions with the fifth dose of vaccine in order to be able to reduce their frequency.

Severe reactions. There are other reactions after pertussis vaccination that cause more concern to parents and physicians than those listed above. Severe reactions that may occur after DTaP vaccine include allergic reactions, prolonged crying, "collapse" reaction, high fever and convulsions [see Table 5.4, below].

A variety of **allergic reactions** have been recorded following DTaP vaccine. Most of these reactions are skin rashes, such as hives. Much less frequently, the child may have swelling of the face or lips, difficulty breathing or wheezing. Severe allergic reactions such as anaphylaxis (which can result in shock or low blood pressure, obstruction of the airways and death) were described as occurring with the first pertussis vaccines in the 1930s.

With vaccines made since the early 1940s, the occurrence of anaphylaxis has been so rare following the vaccine that it is not possible to calculate the risk. Naturally, any child who has an allergic reaction after DTaP or any other vaccine should not receive the same vaccine again until a physician has evaluated the child and identified the cause of the reaction.

About 1 in 300 infants have non-stop, **inconsolable crying** or screaming lasting more than 3 hours after DTaP vaccine. Excessive crying begins within 12 hours of the injection and is thought to be caused by pain and tenderness at the site of a large local reaction. There is no evidence that prolonged crying is caused by irritation of the brain. Permanent brain damage has not been observed in babies who have this reaction. The infants recover completely from the episode.

Another reaction that may frighten parents is the **collapse reaction**, also called a *hypotonic-hyporesponsive episode (HHE)*. The reaction occurs most often after the first dose of DTaP and almost never after the fourth or fifth dose. The frequency of HHE is between once in every 2,100 to 4,200 injections of Canadian vaccines containing DTaP.

Symptoms of HHE. Symptoms begin within 12 hours of the injection and may last up to 1 day. The infant becomes pale, floppy and less responsive than normal. In spite of the infant's appearance, blood pressure remains normal and shock does not occur. Blood sugar also remains normal during the episode.

The cause of HHE is unknown. Infants with collapse reaction recover completely. Death or brain damage has not been recorded in infants having this reaction. Infants who have had the collapse reaction are not at risk of another such episode when given DTaP again.

Fever greater than 40°C (104°F) occurs after about 1 in 3,000 doses in babies who have not been given acetaminophen (Tylenol, Tempra, etc.) at the time of vaccination. (High fever is so uncommon with acellular pertussis vaccine that routine use of acetaminophen is no longer recommended before vaccination.) Fever following DTaP vaccine is never so high that it can cause permanent damage to the brain or any other organ.

Almost 3% of healthy children will have one or more **convulsions with fever**, regardless of the cause of fever. Children who are susceptible to convulsions with fever may have one after vaccination if the vaccination causes fever. DTaP vaccine can induce fever, so some infants may have a convulsion after vaccination. The exact rate of occurrence of convulsions after DTaP is not known, but is somewhere between 1 in 2,900 doses and 1 in 50,000 doses.

A study was done at 12 Canadian children's hospitals of infants hospitalized because of febrile convulsions (those caused by fever) after receiving an injection containing pertussis vaccine. The number of infants hospitalized declined by more than 80% after the introduction of acellular pertussis vaccine.

Convulsions are more common after the third and fourth doses than after the first two doses and are very rare after the fifth dose. As stated above, convulsions associated with DTaP vaccine are caused by fever. Most febrile convulsions occur in children between 6 months and 6 years of age.

Children whose parents or siblings have had convulsions are more likely to have a convulsion with fever than those with no such history. Febrile convulsions do not cause permanent brain damage and do not increase the risk of epilepsy or any other disorder of the brain.

TABLE 5.4

Severe adverse events after DTaP vaccine

REACTION	FREQUENCY	LONG-TERM CONSEQUENCES
Prolonged crying	1 in 300 doses	None
HHE	1 in 2,100 to 4,200 doses	None
High fever, greater than 40°C (104°F)	1 in 3,000 doses	None
Febrile convulsion	1 in 2,900 to 50,000 doses	None
Anaphylaxis	Extremely rare (too rare to calculate)	Can cause death

Claims of other dangers. None of the above severe reactions, other than anaphylaxis (which is extremely rare), causes permanent damage of any kind. There are a great number of other conditions that have been blamed on pertussis vaccine. Most such allegations of the dangers of pertussis vaccine are based on anecdotes (personal stories) and have not been confirmed by scientific studies.

Temporal — not causal — association. Vaccination of infants occurs frequently over a short period of time: most children are vaccinated three times between 2 and 6 months of age. It is quite possible that other unrelated medical problems will occur or be discovered during this period, too. There is a temporal association here — events occur within the same time frame. Unfortunately, there is a tendency to blame the vaccine for every symptom and ailment that develops during this time.

Based on all the reports published and studies performed by reliable sources, *pertussis vaccine* does *not* cause encephalopathy, brain damage, autism, infantile spasms, epilepsy, mental retardation, learning disorders, hyperactivity or sudden infant death syndrome (SIDS). In contrast, based on medical fact, *pertussis infection can* cause pneumonia, convulsions, brain damage and death.

Studies don't support causal relationship. Since no laboratory or other tests exist that can identify pertussis vaccine as the cause of encephalopathy or other rare, severe problems, scientists and researchers can only compare how often the particular condition occurs in vaccinated and unvaccinated children. If the rates are the same for both groups of children, it is very unlikely that the vaccine caused the problem.

Brain dysfunction. Acute encephalopathy is a condition in which a person suddenly develops marked abnormalities of brain function, including some or all of the following: seizures, aggressiveness, psychosis, stupor or coma. There have been many reports in the medical and lay press over the past 60 years of acute encephalopathy following pertussis vaccine. Such reports by themselves provide no evidence of whether pertussis vaccine actually causes the condition.

A study of 54,000 pregnant women was carried out at 12 hospitals in the United States, starting in 1959. Their children's health was monitored until the age of 7. Ten children (1 in every 5,400) had a febrile convulsion within 2 weeks of pertussis vaccination. All 10 were recorded as having normal intelligence and school performance when last examined. There were no cases of acute encephalopathy.

Four other studies in the United States and England involved approximately 415,000 children who received nearly 1 million doses of the combined diphtheria toxoid, whole cell pertussis and tetanus toxoid vaccine (DPT). One of the studies did find that there was an increased risk of convulsions due to fever in the first 3 days after vaccination, but as previously mentioned, such convulsions do not cause brain damage. No cases of encephalopathy or other acute illness involving the brain occurred within 7 days of vaccination.

The National Childhood Encephalopathy Study in the United Kingdom found that there might be a slightly increased risk of acute encephalopathy following pertussis vaccine. However, the study did not provide useful information about the occurrence of permanent brain damage. The scientific information provided by these studies leads to the conclusion that if brain damage ever occurs after pertussis vaccine, it is an extremely rare event: less than 1 in 1 million.

On the basis of these and other scientific studies, expert groups in Canada (Canadian Paediatric Society, National Advisory Committee on Immunization), the United States (American Academy of Pediatrics, Institute of Medicine), the United Kingdom (British Paediatric Association, British Vaccine Injury Compensation Program) and Australia (Australian Pediatric Association) all agree that there is no scientific evidence that pertussis vaccine causes brain damage.

Infantile spasms is another neurologic condition in infants for which pertussis vaccine has been blamed. An estimated 150 infants are affected by this seizure disorder in Canada every year. The seizures are complex and difficult to control. Most children with the disorder are afflicted with permanent handicaps, including cerebral palsy, delayed development and/or mental retardation.

Infantile spasms usually begin between 2 and 8 months of age, the same age span as the scheduled administration of 3 doses of DTaP (2, 4 and

6 months). It should therefore be expected that onset of infantile spasms (an uncommon event) will sometimes coincide with DTaP vaccination (a common event).

Because babies with infantile spasms seem normal in the first few months of life, parents blame an external influence occurring after birth, such as a vaccine. However, brain scans reveal that many children with infantile spasms have malformations of the brain that clearly occurred before birth. Vaccination is not the cause of infantile spasms.

In Denmark before 1970, the first dose of pertussis vaccine was given at 5 months of age. After 1970, the age at which the first dose should be given was lowered to 5 weeks of age. There was no change in the age of onset of infantile spasms following the change in vaccination schedule. The National Childhood Encephalopathy Study in the United Kingdom found that children with infantile spasms were less likely to have received DTaP vaccine or DT (diphtheria and tetanus toxoids without pertussis vaccine) in the 28 days before onset of their illness. These and other studies were unable to find any evidence to suggest that pertussis vaccine causes infantile spasms.

SIDS. Finally, pertussis vaccine has been blamed for many cases of sudden infant death syndrome (SIDS). Over 3,000 infants die of SIDS every year in the United States. Since most of these deaths occur before 6 months of age, it is no surprise that some of the children had been vaccinated shortly before they died.

The association between vaccination and SIDS is purely coincidental. No large-scale scientific study has confirmed an association between SIDS and vaccination. In fact, scientific studies in the United States, England and France found that infants that died of SIDS were *less likely* to have been vaccinated than infants in the control group (infants in the study who didn't die).

In Sweden, no change in the incidence of SIDS was observed following the discontinuation or decrease of pertussis vaccination in 1979.

Similarly, in Japan and England, there was no change in the number of SIDS cases when vaccination rates declined in the 1970s.

In the United States and other countries, the number of SIDS deaths has decreased markedly in the past 4 years even though more children are being vaccinated with pertussis vaccine than ever before. The decrease in cases involving SIDS is due to the success of the "Back to Sleep" campaign, which advises parents to place their babies on their backs for sleeping.

After reviewing all of the available data, the Institute of Medicine in the United States concluded that there is no causal relation between DTaP vaccine and death from SIDS or death from any other cause.

Critics of vaccination often claim that pertussis vaccine is the cause of many other conditions including *autism, behaviour disorders, learning disorders, hyperactivity, AIDS, cancer, leukemia* and almost every other illness affecting children. There are no data to support any of these claims.

Furthermore, there is no known way that pertussis vaccine could produce such effects. [For more information, see reports issued by the Institute of Medicine at www.iom.edu/iom/iomhome.nsf/Pages/immunization+safety+review. See also Chapter 2.]

Reasons to Avoid or Delay Pertussis Vaccine

Do not give. The National Advisory Committee on Immunization recognizes only one absolute reason not to give pertussis vaccine: an anaphylactic reaction to a previous dose of the vaccine. Anaphylaxis is a severe allergic reaction involving one or more of the following: swelling of face or lips, difficulty breathing or shock (fall in blood pressure).

Do not delay. Vaccination should not be deferred or delayed because of minor illnesses, such as the common cold, with or without fever. Such infections do not increase the risk of side effects and do not interfere with the immune response to vaccination.

Delay. Moderate to severe illness, with or without fever, is a reason to delay routine immunization. This precaution should be taken to avoid adding any side effects of the vaccine on top of the effects of the illness itself. However, if pertussis is occurring in the community, vaccination is recommended because the risk of pertussis in an unimmunized infant is much greater than the risk of any side effects.

The Results of Vaccination

Great success with acellular vaccine. Routine use of acellular pertussis vaccine has had great benefits. The efficacy (production of a desired result) of acellular pertussis vaccine has been demonstrated in a number of ways.

Controlled research trials comparing the frequency of disease in vaccinated and unvaccinated children have shown that the Canadian acellular pertussis vaccine protected 85% of vaccinated children against severe illness, defined as coughing spells lasting 21 days or more.

It was equally effective in preventing mild illness. The vaccine does not always prevent infection, but the illness is much milder in those who become infected in spite of being vaccinated.

A marked decline in cases. Routine vaccination of infants and young children has resulted in a marked decline in the frequency of pertussis in every country in which vaccination programs have been introduced. It is true that the *number of infant deaths* from pertussis declined in Canada, the United States and Western Europe long before pertussis vaccine was available; however, no decline in the *number of cases* occurred before mass vaccination began.

Outbreaks in other countries. The benefit of routine vaccination against pertussis has also been confirmed by the experiences in Japan, Sweden, England, Wales and Russia. Routine pertussis vaccination began in *Japan* in 1950. Before that time, there were over 100,000 cases every year. By 1974, the number had decreased to about 200–400 per year. In 1975, use of pertussis vaccine was halted in Japan following the deaths of two infants who had received DPT, which contained whole cell (not acellular) pertussis vaccine.

The ban against pertussis vaccine was lifted 2 months later when the deaths were judged as having been caused by something other than the vaccine. But many parents still refused to have their children vaccinated; they were frightened by the publicity surrounding the deaths. The vaccination rate fell from 90% to less than 40%.

In the 4 years before the temporary ban, there were only 400 cases and 2 to 3 deaths per year from pertussis. After the ban and the ensuing drop in the vaccination rate, an epidemic of pertussis occurred between 1976 and 1979 in Japan, with over 13,000 cases and more than 100 deaths. Following the introduction of routine immunization with acellular pertussis, the rates of pertussis in Japan returned to levels similar to those seen prior to 1974.

In *Sweden*, use of pertussis vaccine (made in Sweden) was discontinued in 1979 because of concern regarding its efficacy and safety. Soon after, the number of cases of pertussis increased markedly: the rate of pertussis became 10 times higher in Sweden than in Canada. Over 60% of children in Sweden got pertussis by 10 years of age. After routine immunization against pertussis was started again in the 1990s, using acellular pertussis vaccine, the frequency of pertussis declined dramatically.

Prior to 1970, the rate of pertussis was very low in *England and Wales* because of high rates of immunization. However, following news stories in the early 1970s of the alleged dangers of pertussis vaccine, vaccination rates there declined from 75% to about 25% by 1975.

Two large epidemics of pertussis occurred between 1977 and 1979 and 1981 and 1982. There were over 100 deaths from pertussis during the first outbreak. When occurrence rates in different parts of the United

Kingdom were compared, areas with low rates of vaccination had high rates of pertussis, and vice versa. Once immunization rates increased — following scientific studies of side effects and extensive public education — the rates of pertussis again declined to very low levels.

A very similar experience occurred in *Russia* following widespread publicity about the alleged dangers of pertussis vaccine: vaccination rates dropped and the rates of pertussis increased to the highest levels recorded among developed countries.

Protection — effective but not long-lasting. Protection provided by acellular pertussis vaccine may not last very long. In fact, studies in England following use of the older whole cell pertussis vaccine suggest that immunity may be gone within 3 to 5 years after the last dose of vaccine. Such loss of immunity would explain why pertussis is so common in adolescents and young adults. Studies in Canada, the United States and Australia have shown that 20–25% of young adults with a cough lasting more than 1 week have pertussis, in spite of having been vaccinated in early childhood.

The large number of pertussis cases among teenagers and young adults explains why the disease continues to be with us in spite of widespread vaccination of infants and young children. The newly developed booster for adolescents and adults will provide longer lasting protection.

Benefits of protection. The major benefit of acellular pertussis vaccine is that it reduces the severity of illness and risk of complications. Since the risk of complications from the disease is highest in infants less than 6 months of age, it is very important to begin vaccination as early as possible, which is at 2 months of age.

Evidence that pertussis vaccine works includes:
- the marked decline of pertussis cases and related deaths in all countries in which immunization of infants and children is routine;
- the occurrence of epidemics of pertussis in Japan, Sweden, England, Wales and Russia after marked falls in immunization rates followed by control of the outbreaks with mass immunization;

- an 85% reduction of the number of cases in fully immunized children during controlled studies of acellular pertussis vaccine;
- milder disease and fewer complications in fully immunized persons.

Summary

- All infants and young children should receive pertussis vaccine.
- Pertussis is a severe disease in young infants. About 1 in 400 infants with pertussis dies and 1 in 400 suffers permanent brain damage from pertussis.
- Complications of pertussis (such as ear infections and pneumonia) are common. Even without complications, infants are sick for 3 to 12 weeks.
- Pertussis vaccine does not prevent infection in everyone. However, it is very effective in reducing the severity of illness and the risk of complications.
- Pertussis is much less common in countries with programs of routine vaccination of all infants.
- Minor side effects are common with the current vaccine. There is no evidence that pertussis vaccine causes permanent brain damage, SIDS, developmental delay, autism, attention deficit disorder, behaviour disorders, learning disorders, hyperactivity, AIDS, cancer or leukemia, or any other severe or chronic condition.
- Parents can consider using acellular pertussis vaccine to protect their adolescent children (and themselves) if they are willing to pay for the vaccine.

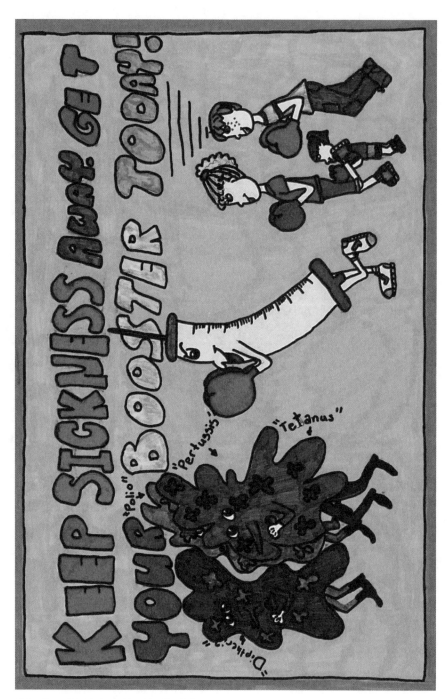

Robyn Reynolds, Manuels, Newfoundland

CHAPTER 6

Polio

Polio (short for poliomyelitis) is an infection caused by a virus called poliovirus. Most infections with poliovirus occur without any noticeable illness. However in its most severe form, poliovirus can infect and destroy certain nerve cells in the spinal cord that control the contraction of muscles. When the nerve cells die, the muscles become weak or paralyzed. The nerve damage is permanent.

A History of Polio

Before Vaccine

A global disease. Before the polio vaccine became available, paralytic polio was the most common infectious cause of major crippling disease.

Polio occurred worldwide — year-round in the tropics, and during the summer and fall in temperate regions. Until about 100 years ago, almost all infants became infected with polio. However, the infection rarely resulted in paralytic polio because the infants were partly protected by antibodies passed on to them from their mothers.

Urban epidemics. In the late 19th and early 20th centuries in North America and Western Europe, epidemics of paralytic polio began to occur in urban areas. As most children were not immune, the virus flourished whenever it was introduced into a community. Fortunately, improved sanitation and hygiene reduced the risk of exposure to poliovirus for infants and young children. But when older children and adults encountered poliovirus, the infection was more likely to result in paralytic disease than in infants.

Last major epidemics in North America. Between 1951 and 1954, just before polio vaccine became available, there were over 65,000 cases of paralytic polio in the United States. The last major epidemic in Canada occurred in 1959, with nearly 2,000 cases of paralytic polio. During that outbreak, the rate of paralytic disease was highest in children 5 to 9 years of age. However paralytic polio does also occur in adolescents and adults: over one-third of cases in Canada and the United States have involved persons over the age of 15.

After Vaccine

A significant reduction in cases. In 1955, a total of more than 76,000 cases of paralytic polio were reported in Canada, the United States, the former Soviet Union, Western Europe, Australia and New Zealand. In 1967, there were only 1,013 cases in these same countries — a reduction of almost 99% in just 12 years.

Continued reductions in the frequency of paralytic polio occurred in all countries with successful polio vaccination programs. The last case of paralytic polio due to wild poliovirus in the United States occurred in 1980, and in Canada in 1989. (Strains of poliovirus that cause disease are referred to as wild poliovirus; the strains of virus in polio vaccines are called vaccine strains.)

The global campaign to eradicate polio, promoted by UNICEF and the World Health Organization, has been remarkably successful. In 1988, the World Health Organization estimated that 350,000 cases of paralytic polio had occurred that year. By 1999, the number had been reduced to 20,000, a decrease of 94%!

Poliovirus has been eradicated from the entire Western Hemisphere: the last known case of disease due to wild virus occurred in Peru in September 1991. Poliovirus has also been eradicated from Western Europe, Australia, New Zealand, Japan, China, Indonesia, and the other countries of Southeast Asia.

Not yet 100%. Polioviruses still are being spread and causing paralytic disease in South Asia (India, Pakistan, Bangladesh, Afghanistan and Nepal) and parts of Africa. Because wild poliovirus, like smallpox, infects only humans, it can be eradicated if all children are vaccinated.

With National Immunization Days [for more detail, see *The results of vaccination* later in this chapter] — vaccination programs that take place in developing countries — global eradication is quite possible in the next few years. Until the virus has been eliminated worldwide, children must continue to be immunized in Canada. The risk of travellers bringing polioviruses back into Canada is too great to ignore.

The Germ

How It Causes Illness

Paralytic polio is caused by infection with poliovirus. The virus was first grown in the laboratory in 1949. There are three different types of poliovirus: types 1, 2 and 3. The proteins responsible for differences in the three types are located in the external coat of the virus.

Polioviruses attach to a specific protein in the membrane of human cells. This protein is present only in humans, chimpanzees and some monkeys, which explains why polioviruses can infect only humans and these animals. (Although chimps and some monkeys can be infected with polioviruses in the laboratory, polioviruses have not been found in animals in the wild.)

After entering the body, the virus infects cells in the throat and in the intestinal tract. The virus multiplies and then spreads through the blood to the spinal cord and brain. Within the spinal cord, the virus moves along nerve fibres. If a large amount of virus grows in the spinal cord, nerve cells that activate muscles are destroyed. Depending on the extent of nerve cell damage, weakness or complete paralysis of muscles occurs.

How Polio Is Spread

Direct and indirect contact. Poliovirus is found in the throat and feces of infected patients. Infected persons spread the virus in two ways: from the throat directly to another person or from the feces by contamination of water, food or hands.

From the throat. Direct spread of poliovirus requires close contact between people. An infected person may cough or sneeze, spreading droplets containing many virus particles. These particles may land in the nose or throat of another person.

Feces contamination. The virus in the feces can spread because of poor hygiene and inadequate sanitation. An infected person who does not wash his or her hands properly after going to the bathroom can spread the virus directly by touching other persons, or indirectly by contaminating food, water and objects. Inadequate sewage treatment can lead to contamination of the environment, especially the water supply. If the water supply is contaminated, the virus can spread to many people.

Contagious. The spread of polio was a mystery until it was discovered that only 1 out of 100 infected persons develops paralytic disease. Until that time, researchers were unaware that there were 99 others who had mild illness or no illness at all. This explained the rapid spread of infection.

All infected persons are contagious, regardless of severity of their illness. Virus is shed from the throat for 1 to 2 weeks after infection, and from the intestines for 4 to 8 weeks afterwards.

The Illness

Symptoms. The time between infection and the start of symptoms is usually 7 to 14 days. About 90–95% of infected persons have no symptoms at all after infection. The only sign of infection in another 4–8% of persons is a minor illness lasting a few days. Symptoms may include one or more of the following: fever, sore throat, muscle aches and pains, drowsiness, headache, loss of appetite, nausea, vomiting, abdominal pain and constipation.

In 1–5% of patients, symptoms indicating spread of virus to the spinal cord and/or brain develop 1 to 2 days later. This form of the infection is called viral or aseptic meningitis. The patient has stiffness of the neck, severe headache, vomiting, and lethargy or drowsiness because the virus has invaded and caused inflammation of the membranes and fluid covering the brain and spinal cord. The illness lasts 2 to 10 days, followed by rapid and complete recovery.

Severe illness. Only about 1 out of every 100 persons infected with the virus gets the severe form of the disease, *paralytic polio*. Sudden onset of weakness or paralysis of muscles occurs in various parts of the body. Often there is severe pain in non-paralyzed muscles. The degree to which a person will be paralyzed is reached within a few days.

Recovery of muscle function may occur, but most patients are permanently paralyzed.

The paralysis usually affects one part of the body more than others. Paralysis of the leg is much more common than paralysis of the arm. A few patients may have paralysis of the diaphragm and chest muscles, leading to reduced ability or complete inability to breathe. Such patients require artificial mechanical ventilators to survive.

Complications

Death from paralytic polio can occur in severe cases as a result of damage to nerve centres controlling respiration, circulation and other vital functions. Patients who require a mechanical ventilator to breathe because of paralysis of muscles necessary for respiration are at increased risk of acquiring pneumonia, which may cause death.

Post-polio syndrome. Some people who have had paralytic polio have reported experiencing a progression of muscle pain, weakness and paralysis — a condition called post-polio syndrome. The interval between the original illness and the onset of new symptoms may be as long as 15 to 40 years.

Possibly one-quarter of patients with paralytic polio may develop post-polio syndrome. It is not possible for the virus to cause the progressive muscle disease, as the virus no longer exists in the person. This disorder probably results from the effects of overuse or aging of damaged muscles.

Diagnosis

Diagnosis of polio is based on the results of cultures (growing the virus from the feces or spinal fluid) obtained during the first 2 weeks after onset of paralysis. Blood tests to detect an increase in specific antibody to poliovirus may also aid in the diagnosis, but are less useful than cultures.

Treatment

Supportive treatments. There are no drugs that cure polio or relieve paralysis. Supportive treatments (warm baths, massage and physiotherapy) help relieve the muscle pain during the acute illness and prevent complications caused by muscle paralysis. Ventilators enable those with paralysis of respiratory muscles to breathe. Long-term care and rehabilitation can help the patient cope with disability.

Post-recovery. As with most infections, immunity develops after infection and repeat attacks of paralytic polio are extremely rare.

The Vaccine

Types of Vaccines

There are two different kinds of polio vaccine: inactivated polio vaccine (IPV), which contains killed, intact virus; and oral polio vaccine (OPV), which contains live, attenuated (weakened) virus. Both vaccines contain the three polioviruses, types 1, 2 and 3. Only IPV is used in Canada and the United States now. [For details on why use of OPV was discontinued, see below, *Possible side effects of polio vaccines.*]

IPV — killed, intact virus. IPV contains only dead virus and cannot cause paralytic polio.

OPV — live, attenuated virus. OPV, the kind of vaccine used prior to 1997–98 in British Columbia, Alberta, Saskatchewan, Manitoba, Quebec and New Brunswick, contains live strains of the three types of poliovirus, which have been weakened in the laboratory.

The vaccine strains have undergone changes that greatly reduce their ability to damage nerve cells without affecting their ability to infect cells in the throat and intestinal tract. The desired result: the vaccine strains can cause an infection and stimulate an immune response without causing a full-blown case of polio.

Because the oral, weakened vaccine strains have not *completely* lost the ability to cause damage to nerve cells, there is a very small risk of getting paralytic polio after receiving OPV [see below, *Possible side effects of polio vaccines*].

How Polio Vaccines Are Made

Growing virus in the laboratory. Viruses can grow only inside cells. This is why vaccines against infections caused by viruses such as polio, measles, mumps and rubella could not be made until a method was discovered for growing animal or human cells in test tubes or flasks.

In the 1950s, Dr. John Enders and his colleagues developed a method called tissue culture. They added live ("wild") poliovirus to the cells in a test tube and found that the virus infected the cells and multiplied inside them. The new virus could then be extracted from the cells and purified. The new method enabled them to grow large amounts of poliovirus in the laboratory for the first time. They were awarded the Nobel Prize for this research.

Large quantities of wild poliovirus are now grown within cells in very large containers instead of test tubes!

Process for making IPV. This vaccine is produced using either specific human cells (MRC-5 cells) or Vero cells derived from monkeys. The MRC-5 cells were derived from cells taken from a single fetus decades ago. The Vero cells were derived from monkeys born and raised in special breeding facilities. The cells are stored in freezers until they are needed. All of the cells used to make polio vaccines today have been studied for many years. They are tested repeatedly to make sure that no contaminating viruses are present.

The poliovirus particles are separated from the cells, purified and concentrated. The fluid is filtered and then treated with formaldehyde to kill (inactivate) the virus. (The vaccine contains less than 30 parts per million of formaldehyde after the inactivation process.) The final product contains all three types of killed poliovirus.

Additives to IPV. Antibiotics are added during the manufacturing process to prevent contamination by bacteria. During purification, the antibiotics are reduced to barely detectable levels. The dose of each type is adjusted and a preservative (phenoxyethanol) is added.

The vaccine does *not* contain thimerosal, a mercury-containing preservative. In fact, thimerosal *cannot be used* as a preservative for vaccines containing IPV because it damages the vaccine.

Testing of IPV. Each batch of vaccine is tested many times to ensure that no live poliovirus is present. Each batch is also tested for potency (effectiveness) by comparing it with a standard vaccine supplied by the World Health Organization. The vaccine can safely be stored for at least 2 years when refrigerated at 5–8°C (41–46°F).

Process for making OPV. This vaccine is a mixture of the three types of attenuated or weakened live poliovirus, each grown separately in monkey kidney cells and then mixed. The cells are derived from monkeys born and raised in special breeding facilities. As with IPV, all of the cells used to make oral polio vaccines are tested repeatedly to make sure that no contaminating viruses are present.

The monkey kidney cells used to produce polio vaccines are first grown (multiplied) in fluid containing amino acids, salts, calf serum and antibiotics. (Calf serum is added because it was found to be necessary for growth of the cells.) After the cells have completed their growth, the fluid is removed and replaced with fresh fluid *without* calf serum. The attenuated poliovirus is then added.

All manufacturers of OPV start with vaccine strains provided by the World Health Organization and then weaken them. Attenuation or weakening of a virus involves repeated infections of cells in tissue culture. Each time the virus multiplies, mutations may occur in the cell's genes. After many infections, strains of the virus are tested in animals to determine whether the virus has changed in the desired way.

An attenuated virus vaccine must be able to cause an infection, but no longer cause damage. Once such a strain has been isolated, large amounts of it are grown and stored for future production of vaccine.

Additives to OPV. After the three types of viruses have grown in the cells, they are separated from the fluid culture and diluted with fluid containing sorbitol (a sugar alcohol) as a stabilizer. All three types of viruses are mixed in the appropriate concentrations to make the final product. Each dose of vaccine contains very small amounts of the antibiotics streptomycin and neomycin (less than 25 μg each, or 0.000025 g).

Testing of OPV. The vaccines are tested for safety by injection into monkeys; the animals are then examined for evidence of nerve cell damage. Each lot of vaccine must be shown to be as safe as a standard vaccine lot supplied by the World Health Organization. Although OPV contains live viruses, it retains effectiveness for many years when stored frozen.

Available Forms of Polio Vaccine

Combinations. In Canada, IPV is supplied either alone or in combination with the following vaccines:
- DTaP (diphtheria and tetanus toxoids and acellular pertussis vaccine);
- DT (diphtheria and tetanus toxoids);
- Td (tetanus and lower-dose diphtheria vaccine for children aged 7 and over and adults).

The combination DTaP/IPV vaccine (a liquid) can be used to dissolve the *Haemophilus influenzae* type b (Hib) vaccine (a powder) so that all five vaccines can be administered as a single injection.

Vaccines for older children and adults. There is no lower-dose polio vaccine for children aged 7 and over and adults.

How the Vaccine Is Given

IPV is administered by injection into muscle. In Canada, it is usually given in combination with DTaP and Hib vaccines as a single injection.

IPV, whether alone or in combination with other vaccines, is supplied in a volume of 0.5 ml (one-tenth of a teaspoon). Vaccines are administered by injection into muscle. In infants (children less than 12 months old), the vaccine is usually injected into the thigh because the muscle there is relatively large. In older children, the vaccine is usually given in the muscle of the upper arm.

It is important that vaccines are injected into the muscle rather than into the overlying tissue beneath the skin (subcutaneous tissue). Injection into muscle causes much milder local reaction (e.g., redness, swelling) than injection under the skin.

OPV is given by mouth, and children like the taste of it.

Schedule of Vaccination

Infants and children (under age 7). To achieve long-lasting protection, IPV is administered as a series of injections. When combined with DTaP, it is given at 2, 4 and 6 months of age, with boosters at 18 months and 4 to 6 years of age. If a dose is missed or delayed for any reason, the series does not have to be started again.

Children (age 7 and over) and adults. The schedule for older children and adults is 2 doses of IPV, administered 6 to 8 weeks apart, followed by a booster 6 to 12 months later.

Boosters (to enhance prior vaccinations). Additional doses of IPV are not needed by adolescents or adults who have been fully immunized.

Duration of protection. Protection is long-lasting.

Possible Side Effects of Polio Vaccines

Side effects of IPV. This vaccine is very safe. It is the only polio vaccine used in Canada; OPV has not been used since 1997-98. Other than minor pain and redness at the injection site, side effects after IPV are extremely rare. Current methods of production and testing before releasing the vaccine for use ensure that there is no live virus in the vaccine. Consequently, there have been no cases of paralytic disease resulting from use of IPV produced since 1955.

Risks associated with OPV. Attenuation of strains of poliovirus used in OPV greatly reduces their ability to cause nerve damage. Compared with the wild virus strain, safety tests show that OPV reduces the risk of damage in monkey spinal cords by a factor of at least 1 million. Nevertheless, the potential to cause nerve damage is still present.

The risk of vaccine-associated paralytic polio is estimated to be 1 case in 750,000 first doses of vaccine and 1 case in 6.9 million subsequent doses. The risk for those in very close contact with an infant vaccinated with OPV is 1 case in over 20 million doses of vaccine.

Although the risk of paralytic disease after OPV is extremely low (there have been no cases of vaccine-associated paralytic polio since 1955 with OPV), there is no reason to take the risk because IPV is equally effective and is risk-free.

SV40 discovered in IPV and OPV. In 1960, researchers discovered that some rhesus monkey kidney cells used to grow poliovirus were infected with another virus called simian virus 40, or SV40. It was then found that SV40 causes a "silent" infection in rhesus monkeys in their natural habitat. The virus remained in the kidney cells of wild monkeys without causing any damage, but began to multiply when the cells were grown in laboratory cultures.

When batches of both IPV and OPV were tested, they were found to contain live SV40. Treatment with formaldehyde, which killed poliovirus, did not kill all of the SV40. Once SV40 was identified, steps were taken to ensure that all cells used to grow poliovirus were free of SV40.

Vaccines now SV40-free. Since 1963, all polio vaccines must be tested and shown to be free of SV40 before they can be used. Therefore, SV40 is not an issue for anyone who has been immunized since then.

SV40 studies. SV40 is a member of a group of viruses called papovaviruses, which are known to cause cancer in several species of animals. Two studies have examined whether there were any harmful consequences in persons who received IPV or OPV that contained SV40. The first study found no differences in the death rate (from all causes or from cancer) among groups who had received vaccine that contained SV40 compared with those given vaccine free of SV40.

A second study followed approximately 1,000 infants who had received OPV containing SV40 and 150 who had received IPV with SV40 in it. These children were monitored for 17 to 19 years. No increase in the occurrence of cancer or death (due to cancer or any other cause) was found. This evidence suggests that it is highly unlikely that SV40 causes cancer or any other disease in humans.

Reasons to Avoid or Delay Polio Vaccine

Do not give. The National Advisory Committee on Immunization recognizes only one absolute reason not to give IPV vaccine: an anaphylactic reaction to a previous dose of the vaccine. Anaphylaxis is a severe allergic reaction involving one or more of the following: swelling of face or lips, difficulty breathing or shock (fall in blood pressure). Such reactions are very rare.

Do not delay. Vaccination should not be deferred or delayed because of minor illnesses, such as the common cold, with or without fever. Such infections do not increase the risk of side effects and do not interfere with the immune response to vaccination.

Delay. Moderate to severe illness, with or without fever, is a reason to delay routine immunization. This precaution should be taken to avoid adding any side effects of the vaccine on top of the effects of the illness itself.

The Results of Vaccination

IPV

Effective and long-lasting. After 3 doses of IPV, 100% of infants develop protective levels of antibodies against all three types of poliovirus. The boosters given at 18 months and between 4 and 6 years of age ensure that protective antibodies persist in 100% of recipients for many years.

High levels of protection. Field trials of the original IPV (Salk vaccine) produced between 1955 and 1959 showed that it protected against paralytic polio in 55% of recipients after 1 dose, 80% after 2 doses, 91% after 3 doses, and 96% after 4 doses. Current vaccines are much stronger than the original Salk vaccine and have been shown to be 90% effective after just 2 doses; 100% protection is achieved after the 5 doses recommended in Canada. Protection lasts for many years following vaccination with IPV.

Prevention of outbreaks. The experience in Sweden, Finland, the Netherlands, Iceland and some Canadian provinces (Ontario, Nova Scotia and Newfoundland) has demonstrated that paralytic polio can be eliminated by the use of IPV alone.

Over the past 50 years, travellers infected with polio have brought the virus back into these countries/provinces many times; however only three small outbreaks of paralytic polio have occurred in that time. All cases involved small groups of people who had refused immunization for religious reasons. Although many people came in close contact with infected individuals, no disease occurred in those who had been vaccinated.

OPV

Effective but discontinued. OPV is just as effective as IPV in preventing paralytic disease. Until recently, OPV was used in many countries, including the United States, and in several provinces in Canada (British Columbia, Alberta, Saskatchewan, Manitoba, Quebec and New Brunswick). [For reasons why it was discontinued, see the Text Box earlier in this Chapter.]

Mass vaccination programs in developing countries. Because OPV is less expensive and easier to administer, it has been used extensively in developing countries. The approach to eradication of poliovirus has been to vaccinate all children under 5 years of age in these countries with OPV on the same day. A second dose of OPV is given 4 to 6 weeks later, again on the same day. By vaccinating all young children twice within a very short period, it is possible to overcome the interference caused by other intestinal virus infections.

These mass vaccination programs, promoted by UNICEF and the World Health Organization, are called *National Immunization Days*. Money to buy the OPV vaccine for these programs has been provided by Rotary International. National Immunization Days have proven to be very successful and have been critical to the strategy to eradicate polio worldwide.

IPV and OPV

Evidence that polio vaccine works includes the following:
• Large-scale, controlled field trials of both IPV and OPV demonstrated that both vaccines prevent infection with wild polio virus, thereby preventing paralytic disease.
• Wild poliovirus has been eradicated from the Western Hemisphere and paralytic polio has been markedly reduced elsewhere as a result of vaccination.
• The only cases of paralytic polio in Sweden, Finland, the Netherlands, Iceland and some Canadian provinces (Ontario, Nova Scotia and Newfoundland) over the past 50 years have occurred among small groups of unvaccinated individuals.

Summary

• Both IPV and OPV are very effective in preventing paralytic polio and in eliminating transmission of wild poliovirus.
• IPV is safer in that it contains no live virus.
• Usage of OPV was discontinued in 1997-98 in the United States and in those Canadian provinces that used it rather than IPV.

- Paralytic polio has been eradicated from the Western Hemisphere, Western Europe, Australia, New Zealand, Japan, China, Indonesia, and the other countries of Southeast Asia.
- With the implementation of National Immunization Days, prospects are very good for global eradication by 2005.
- Until worldwide eradication of polio has been achieved, routine polio vaccination of all children should continue.

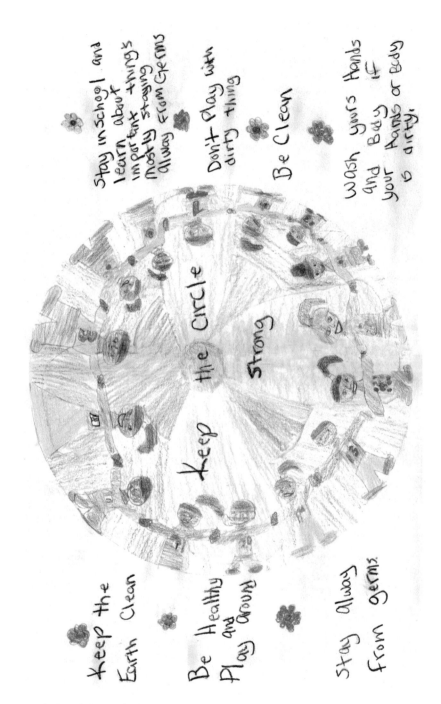

Stay in school and learn about important things Mostly staying alway From Germs

Don't Play with dirty thing

Be Clean

Wash yours Hands and Body if your Aqnds or Body is dirty.

Keep the Circle Strong

Keep the Earth Clean

Be Healthy and Play Around

Stay alway From germs.

Carol Niptayok, Kugaaruk, Nunavut

CHAPTER 7

Haemophilus influenzae type b (Hib)

Haemophilus influenzae type b (or Hib) causes bacterial meningitis and other serious infections. Meningitis is an infection of the membranes and fluid that cover the brain and spinal cord. Hib can also infect the epiglottis (in the throat), blood, lungs, joints, bones and skin. The risk of Hib disease in older children and adults is very low.

In spite of its name, *Haemophilus influenzae* has nothing to do with influenza (the flu), which is caused by a virus, not by bacteria. The bacteria were named *Haemophilus influenzae* because they were incorrectly thought to be the cause of influenza. For convenience and to prevent confusion with influenza, the bacteria are commonly called Hib.

A History of Hib

Before Vaccine

Before 1985, Hib was the most common cause of bacterial meningitis in children in Canada and most other parts of the world. Every year in Canada, about 1,500 cases of Hib meningitis occurred in children under 5 years of age. There were an equal number of other kinds of severe Hib infections in children. About one-half of Hib infections occurred in children less than 18 months old, the majority of whom were 6 to 11 months of age. About 1 in every 300 Canadian children developed meningitis or other severe Hib infections by age 5. It is thought that as many as one-third of all cases of serious pneumonia (an infection of the lungs) in infants were caused by Hib before Hib vaccine became available.

After Vaccine

The first vaccine developed against Hib was tested in Finland in the 1970s and was found to protect children over 2 years of age. Unfortunately, it did not protect the majority of victims of this illness — children less than 2 years old. This vaccine was licensed in Canada in 1986 and was recommended for use in children 2 to 5 years of age. Subsequent research led to improved versions of the vaccine, which were effective in young infants as well.

Hib infections have almost disappeared in countries that have introduced routine immunization of infants with Hib vaccine, such as Canada, the United States, Finland, Iceland, Sweden, the United Kingdom, Germany, France and the Netherlands. In 1985, 485 children with Hib infections were admitted to 10 children's hospitals in Canada. By 2000, only 4 children with Hib disease were admitted to these hospitals — a decrease of 99.2%! Similar remarkable results have been seen in every country with an effective children's immunization program that includes Hib vaccine.

The Germ

How It Causes Illness

Infection of the bloodstream. Hib bacteria infect only humans. Infection starts in the nose or throat where the bacteria attach to the cells lining the surface. If the infected person has no immunity against Hib, the bacteria may invade the bloodstream. Once Hib gets into the bloodstream, it can infect almost any other part of the body, such as the lungs, heart, joints, bones and skin.

Meningitis results when the bacteria infect the fluid and covering of the brain and spinal cord. In some children, a severe infection called epiglottitis occurs in the throat. Marked swelling of the epiglottis (the epiglottis closes off the windpipe when a person swallows) and surrounding structures develops rapidly. The child may suffocate without emergency treatment.

Obstruction of blood vessels. The blood supply to the brain can be affected by inflammation and obstruction of blood vessels. Since brain cells cannot withstand interruption of their blood supply for very long, inflammation can result in permanent brain damage.

How Hib bacteria work. Hib bacteria have an external coat, called the capsule, which is made of a large, complex sugar or *polysaccharide*. The capsule protects the bacteria against attack by the white blood cells, the body's main defence against infection. In someone who lacks antibodies to Hib, the white blood cells are unable to attack and kill Hib bacteria. Therefore, the bacteria can invade the body and multiply freely.

While the capsule protects Hib bacteria from attack by white blood cells, another substance in the wall of the Hib bacteria, called *endotoxin*, causes the damage. Endotoxin is a complex chemical present in many different bacteria. When it is released in the body, it causes an intense reaction, called inflammation. If the bacterial infection is not treated, the inflammation can get out of control and cause damage throughout the body, especially to blood vessels.

How Hib Is Spread

Direct contact, oral contact and contaminated objects. Spread of Hib requires close, direct contact between people. An infected person may cough or sneeze, releasing a spray of droplets containing many bacteria. These bacteria may land in the nose or throat of another person. Hib can also spread by oral contact, such as kissing or sharing drinks. Hib bacteria can survive outside the body for a number of hours; therefore, spread may also occur by touching contaminated objects (e.g., toys shared between children).

Hib infections are **not highly contagious**. It may seem that Hib would be more contagious than diphtheria because the ways in which the bacteria can be spread are more numerous, but this is not so. Someone sick with diphtheria has many more bacteria in the nose and throat and spreads more into the air and immediate environment than someone sick with Hib, pneumococcal or meningococcal disease.

Healthy carriers. Healthy people can be carriers of Hib bacteria. The bacteria can persist and multiply on the surface of the nose or throat without causing any symptoms in someone who has already developed immunity to Hib. Young infants and adults are not often found to be carriers of Hib. Most healthy carriers are toddlers aged 18 to 35 months, and preschool children 3 to 5 years of age.

Prior to routine use of vaccines against Hib, most children became infected with Hib bacteria at least once during the first 5 years of life, usually by contact with other young children (either an older sibling or classmates in day care or preschool programs).

The Illness

Symptoms. The incubation period of Hib disease is not known. Illness probably occurs within a few days of becoming infected. Symptoms can come on suddenly (in a matter of a few hours) or more gradually (over a few days). [Symptoms of various Hib-related infections are described in more detail below.]

Infections. Hib can cause a variety of infections, ranging from mild to severe.

1. The most common is infection of the nose and throat without any illness, called *asymptomatic infection* or colonization. People do not seek treatment because they do not feel ill.

2. *Surface infections* involve the spread of Hib bacteria along the surface (the mucosa) of the respiratory tract, without invading the bloodstream. Surface spread can lead to
   - *otitis* (ear infection),
   - *sinus infections,*
   - *conjunctivitis* (eye infection),
   - *bronchitis* (infection of the airways),
   - *pneumonia* (lung infection).

   There are many other causes for each of these infections. Hib causes only a very small proportion of each type of infection. Therefore, Hib vaccine won't prevent typical ear infections. The most common causes of ear infections are pneumococcus, other strains of *Haemophilus influenzae* (not type b), and bacteria called *Moraxella*.

   Symptoms of surface infections. Surface infections can produce a variety of symptoms, depending on the part of the body affected [see Table 7.1, below, for a summary]. Fever, loss of appetite, nausea, vomiting and other general symptoms may or may not be present.

3. *Invasion of the bloodstream.* This third type of Hib infection is the least common, but most severe. It leads to infections such as
   - *meningitis* (infection of the membranes and fluid that cover the brain and spinal cord),
   - *bacteremia* (infection of the bloodstream),
   - *epiglottitis* (infection of the epiglottis),
   - *osteomyelitis and septic arthritis* (joint and bone infection).

Symptoms of invasive infections. Once Hib bacteria invade the bloodstream, a fever will likely develop. Other symptoms are usually present such as aches and pains, irritability, and a general sense of feeling unwell.

- The earliest signs of *meningitis* are fever and a change in consciousness or behaviour [see Table 7.2]. Fever occurs because of bacteremia. Disturbance of brain function results from changes in the blood supply to the brain. Once the fluid and membranes covering the brain and spinal cord become infected, the blood vessels going to and from the brain become inflamed. The damaged blood vessels narrow or become blocked, interfering with normal blood flow to the brain.

- *Bacteremia* (infection of the bloodstream) usually leads to alterations of blood circulation. Endotoxin [see *How Hib bacteria work*, earlier in this chapter] from Hib bacteria affects blood vessels throughout the body, including the heart itself. Circulation to the skin is often decreased; the child is pale and cool to the touch in spite of having a fever. Heart rate is increased. In severe cases, bacteremia can lead to shock (a life-threatening fall in blood pressure).

- *Epiglottitis* is an infection of the epiglottis (the flap that covers the opening to the airway at the back of the throat). Infection of the epiglottis and surrounding structures by Hib very rapidly leads to marked swelling of the tissue. The swollen epiglottis obstructs the free flow of air into the lungs. The child has to work much harder to move air in and out of the lungs because of the obstruction. This infection can develop *very* rapidly (within 4 to 8 hours). Treatment requires inserting a tube into the nose or mouth, past the swollen epiglottis, and into the airways so that the child can breathe properly while the infection is being cured with antibiotics.

- *Infection of a joint or of bone* is a complication of invasion of Hib into the bloodstream. Symptoms include sudden onset of fever, pain in the affected joint or bone, decreased movement because of pain and tenderness, redness and swelling.

TABLE 7.1

Symptoms and complications
of surface infections caused by Hib bacteria

INFECTED AREA	RESULTING INFECTION	SYMPTOMS	COMPLICATIONS
Ear	Otitis media	• Fever • Local inflamation • Crying from pain	• Deafness • Chronic ear infection
Sinus	Sinusitis	• Fever • Stuffy nose • Crying from pain	• Infection can spread and cause blindness or brain abscess • Death
Eye	Conjunctivitis	• Fever • Redness, swelling of eyelids • Pus from eye	• Infection can spread and cause blindness or brain abscess • Death
Respiratory tract	Bronchitis	• Fever • Cough	• Pneumonia
Lungs	Pneumonia	• Fever • Cough • Rapid breathing (over 50 breaths per minute in infants; over 40 breaths per minute in children over age 2) • Laboured breathing with grunting and retractions (indrawing of ribs on respiration)	• Empyema (pus surrounding the lung) • Death

TABLE 7.2

Signs and symptoms of Hib meningitis

EARLIEST SIGNS AND SYMPTOMS	LATER SIGNS AND SYMPTOMS

• Fever, usually high
• Significant change in behaviour such as
  - drowsiness, confusion, impaired consciousness, coma
  - irritability, fussiness, crying, agitation
  - fussiness and crying alternating with drowsiness
	• Severe headache*
	• Stiff neck or pain/tenderness on moving neck or back*
	• Bulging fontanelle (soft spot on skull)
	• Vomiting
	• Seizure (convulsion)

* Infants unable to talk may cry or be irritable if this sign/symptom is present.

Complications

Of surface infections. [See Table 7.1, above.]

Of meningitis. Even with early diagnosis and proper treatment, Hib meningitis is a very severe disease: *death* occurs in about 1 out of 20 cases. Without treatment, all children with Hib meningitis die.

Brain damage. Brain cells die quickly if their blood supply is interrupted. Some degree of impairment of the blood supply to the brain occurs in every child with meningitis because of damage to blood vessels and increased pressure within the skull.

About 1 in 3 survivors of Hib meningitis has detectable brain damage, the severity of which varies widely. *Permanent brain damage* is much more likely to occur in children who have coma, seizures, paralysis or other neurologic abnormalities during the acute stage of the illness.

Disabilities resulting from the brain damage may include *developmental delay, speech and language disorders, blindness, epilepsy and paralysis*. Some level of *deafness* occurs in about 15% of survivors; profound (total) deafness occurs in 3–5%.

Children who are behaving normally at the time of discharge from hospital are unlikely to develop signs of brain damage later. They may have minor abnormalities on psychological tests, but there is no impairment of behaviour or performance in school.

Of epiglottitis. The swelling of the epiglottis can become so severe that the airway becomes completely blocked and the child dies of suffocation.

Of bacteremia. In severe cases, bacteremia can lead to shock (a life-threatening fall in blood pressure).

Of joint/bone infection. Permanent damage to joints can occur, especially after infection of the hip joint in infants.

Of other infections. Complications arising from the other kinds of Hib infections depend on the part of the body involved.

Diagnosis

Surface infections. Identification of the specific bacterial cause of ear infections requires special tests that are not routinely available. These tests involve obtaining pus from behind the eardrum. It is also difficult to identify the bacteria causing sinusitis and pneumonia because fluid must be obtained directly from the sinuses or lungs. Throat and nose cultures are not adequate.

Serious invasive infections. Diagnosis is made by the presence of Hib bacteria growing in cultures of the patient's blood, spinal fluid, joint fluid or other infected sites. Diagnosis of meningitis can be confirmed only by performing a lumbar puncture on the patient. A special needle is inserted into the spinal canal in the lower back and a small amount of fluid is removed. The extracted fluid is examined for the presence of bacteria, increased numbers of white blood cells, and changes in the concentration of protein and sugar.

Treatment

Antibiotics. Ear infections, sinusitis and pneumonia suspected to be caused by bacteria are treated with antibiotics. In most cases of ear and sinus infections, the antibiotics can be given by mouth. In children with pneumonia, intravenous antibiotics (given by vein) are sometimes necessary because the child is too ill to take medicine by mouth.

Intravenous treatment. All serious infections caused by Hib must be treated with high doses of intravenous antibiotics. Antibiotic treatment reduces the death rate of Hib meningitis by 95%. Additional treatment (e.g., intravenous fluids) to control fever and seizures may be necessary until the child is able to drink. Treatment of meningitis and other invasive infections is given for at least 7 days.

Family members. When one case of serious Hib disease occurs in a family, there is a chance that Hib bacteria may spread to other household members. To avoid this, all family/household members are prescribed an antibiotic called rifampin, which is taken orally. Rifampin reduces the risk that young children (under the age of 5 years) in the home will acquire Hib infection. If all children under 48 months of age have received Hib vaccine, rifampin is not necessary.

Post-recovery. Children who experience serious Hib infections before their second birthday often do not develop solid immunity and may be at risk of a second episode of Hib disease. Such children should be regarded as unimmunized and should be immunized according to the age-appropriate schedule for unimmunized children [see *Schedule of vaccination*, below]. Children who get Hib disease when they are over 2 years of age develop long-lasting immunity and do not have to be immunized.

The Vaccine

Type of Vaccine

Purified bacterial polysaccharide. Hib vaccine is made of a highly purified chemical extracted from Hib bacteria. A complex sugar called a *polysaccharide* forms the protective capsule or outer coat of the bacteria. As a component of the vaccine, this polysaccharide is used to stimulate immunity. Antibodies made by the immune system attach to the polysaccharides and coat the bacteria. This new coating enables white blood cells to attach to the bacteria and kill them.

How Hib Vaccine Is Made

First attempt. The first successful vaccine against Hib disease was actually made of the purified polysaccharide or complex sugar that forms the outer coat of the bacteria. It was effective, however, only in children over 2 years of age. The immune system of young infants did not respond to the pure polysaccharide.

New method. A new type of vaccine was then developed. The purified polysaccharide was chemically linked to a protein, such as diphtheria toxoid or tetanus toxoid. The combined polysaccharide-protein vaccine, known as a *conjugate vaccine*, worked in young infants.

There are now three different Hib conjugate vaccines approved for use in infants starting at 2 months of age. The vaccines differ in the proteins linked to the polysaccharide. They are equally effective in protecting young infants against Hib disease. The vaccine now used in Canada has tetanus toxoid as the protein and is called *Haemophilus* b tetanus toxoid conjugate vaccine.

Process. Hib bacteria are grown in liquid culture. When growth is complete, the bacteria are removed and the polysaccharide is extracted from the fluid. To make the conjugate vaccine, the various manufacturers use different chemical procedures to bind the purified polysaccharide to the protein. The final material is purified and sterilized by filtration. It is then freeze-dried.

Additives. The vaccine does *not* contain thimerosal, a mercury-containing preservative.

Testing. Mandatory tests for potency (effectiveness), toxicity and sterility are carried out on all lots (batches) of vaccine before they can be distributed [see Chapter 2].

Available Forms of Hib Vaccine

Combinations. Hib conjugate vaccine is available as a freeze-dried product. It can be used on its own, but, in Canada, it is usually combined with diphtheria and tetanus toxoids, and acellular pertussis and inactivated polio vaccines (DTaP/IPV) so that all five vaccines can be given as a single injection.

Vaccines for older children and adults. None [see *Schedule of vaccination*, below].

How the Vaccine Is Given

In Canada, the combined liquid DTaP/IPV is used to dissolve the freeze-dried Hib vaccine, and all five vaccines are given as a single injection.

Into muscle. The Hib vaccine, alone or combined with the DTaP/IPV vaccine, is given by injection into muscle. In infants (children less than 12 months old), the vaccine is usually injected into the thigh because the muscle there is relatively large. In older children, the vaccine is usually given in the muscle of the upper arm.

It is important that vaccine combinations containing alum (such as DTaP/IPV) are injected into the muscle rather than into the overlying tissue beneath the skin (subcutaneous tissue). Injection into muscle causes much milder local reaction (e.g., redness, swelling) than injection under the skin.

Schedule of Vaccination

Infants and toddlers (to age 18 months). The combined DTaP/IPV+Hib vaccine is given at 2, 4 and 6 months of age, with a booster at 15 to 18 months of age.

Children between 18 months and 5 years of age who have *not* received the vaccine may be vaccinated, and need only 1 dose of Hib vaccine for full protection against this disease.

Children over age 5 and adults do not receive the vaccine because the risk of Hib disease in older children and adults is very low.

Boosters (to enhance prior vaccinations) — other than the one following the initial series of vaccinations for infants — are not necessary.

Duration of protection. Following primary immunization in infancy, protective levels persist until the booster is given at 15 to 18 months of age. After this primary booster, protective levels of antibody persist for many years. More importantly, immunization results in the development of immune memory so that the immune system is able to make specific antibody promptly and protect the individual who later comes into contact with Hib bacteria.

Possible Side Effects of Hib Vaccine

Hib vaccines are extremely safe. When given as a separate injection, Hib conjugate vaccines cause local redness and pain in 5–15% of infants. Local reactions are milder and much less common than those seen after the DTaP vaccine.

The addition of the Hib vaccine to DTaP or DTaP/IPV vaccines does not increase the frequency or severity of side effects. Basically, side effects from these other vaccines are the same with or without the Hib vaccine.

Reasons to Avoid or Delay Hib Vaccine

Do not give. The National Advisory Committee on Immunization recognizes only one absolute reason not to give Hib vaccine: an anaphylactic reaction to a previous dose of the vaccine. Anaphylaxis is a severe allergic reaction involving one or more of the following: swelling of face or lips, difficulty breathing or shock (fall in blood pressure). Children who have such an allergic reaction after vaccination should be seen and evaluated by a physician to identify the cause of the reaction.

Do not delay. Vaccination should not be deferred or delayed because of minor illnesses, such as the common cold, with or without fever. Such infections do not increase the risk of side effects and do not interfere with the immune response to vaccination.

Delay. Moderate to severe illness, with or without fever, is a reason to delay routine immunization. This precaution should be taken to avoid adding any side effects of the vaccine on top of the effects of the illness itself.

The Results of Vaccination

As noted above, the occurrence of Hib meningitis, epiglottitis and other severe Hib infections has decreased rapidly in Canada and other countries where infants routinely receive Hib vaccine. Within less than 2 years of the start of routine infant vaccination, Hib disease became a rare occurrence in Canada.

The vaccine protects children in two ways:
• Immunity provided by the vaccine protects children from Hib infection becoming established in the nose and throat. With fewer healthy children carrying Hib bacteria, the spread of Hib is decreased. This occurs only if most children are vaccinated. Vaccination decreases but does not eradicate the bacteria.
• Immunity from the vaccine protects each vaccinated child against invasion of Hib into the blood. The antibodies produced by vaccination help the body's defences kill the bacteria before they can cause any damage.

Evidence that Hib vaccine works includes the following:
• Controlled trials have demonstrated that the vaccine prevents meningitis and other serious Hib infections.
• The frequency of Hib meningitis and other serious Hib infections has declined markedly in all countries that added Hib vaccine to their routine infant immunization program.
• The frequency of Hib meningitis and other serious Hib infections declined by 99% in 12 children's hospitals with active programs to detect all such infections, following the introduction of Hib vaccine in Canada.

Studies confirm that not only is Hib *disease* disappearing, but Hib *bacteria* are also disappearing as a result of routine vaccination. It is not yet clear whether routine vaccination will lead to total eradication of Hib bacteria.

Summary

- Hib infections cause severe illness in children, mainly in those under the age of 5.
- In spite of modern treatment, such infections can result in death or severe disabilities.
- Highly purified vaccines against Hib disease have proven to be very safe and effective.
- Hib disease is disappearing from every country in which all infants are routinely vaccinated with Hib vaccine.

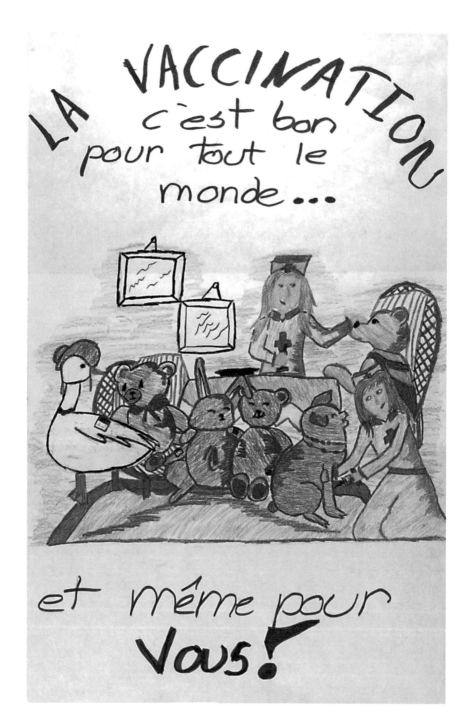

Marie-Claude Thibault, Victoriaville, Quebec

CHAPTER 8

Measles

Measles is a severe illness caused by a virus. It causes high fever, runny nose, cough, conjunctivitis (pink eye or inflammation of the eyelid), and a rash lasting 1 to 2 weeks. It is often complicated by diarrhea, ear infections, croup (a condition resulting from obstruction of the airways) or pneumonia (infection of the lungs).

Encephalitis (intense inflammation of the brain) occurs in about 1 of every 1,000 cases. This condition often results in permanent brain damage. Measles can also cause death. In very rare cases, a severe and always fatal brain disease called SSPE (subacute sclerosing panencephalitis) develops years after the person has had measles.

The first "M" in MMR vaccine stands for measles.

A History of Measles

Before Vaccine

Measles was recognized as a distinct infection in the early 17th century. Most of its features were described by a Danish physician, Peter Panum, during an epidemic on the Faeroe Islands in 1846. He confirmed that measles is contagious and found that the interval between exposure and the start of the rash is 14 days. He also observed that infection results in lifelong immunity: elderly persons living on the islands who had had measles many years before did not get sick during the epidemic.

Measles was found to be a viral infection in 1911, but the virus was not isolated until 1954.

Before vaccine, large epidemics occurred every 2 to 3 years, with the peak being in the late winter and early spring. Measles is highly contagious. Before vaccine, almost everyone got measles by 18 years of age. In Canada, about 300,000 cases occurred every year. Nine out of every 10 cases involved children under 10 years old; more than half of all cases involved children 5 to 9 years old.

The highest risk of complications and death was in children less than 12 months old and in adults. Every year in Canada, measles was responsible for several hundred deaths, 5,000 hospital admissions and 400 cases of encephalitis. The estimated annual cost of measles was over $70 million in 1985 dollars.

After Vaccine

Soon after the measles virus was isolated in 1954, methods were developed to grow the virus in tissue culture cells. Measles vaccine was licensed in 1963. Since then, there has been a dramatic decline in the annual number of cases in every country with routine immunization programs.

Remarkable success. In Canada, the number of cases has fallen more than 99.9%: from an estimated 300,000 per year before 1963 to an average of less than 50 per year since 1998. There has been a similar decline in measles-related deaths and complications such as encephalitis and SSPE [for a detailed description of these two conditions, see *Complications* later in this Chapter]. Before vaccine, there were 50 to 60 cases of SSPE every year in the United States; since 1990, there has been less than 1 case per year.

Through vaccination, many countries have gained remarkable control of measles. Spread of measles virus has been eliminated from Finland and most islands in the Caribbean. Most cases occurring in Canada and the United States since 1998 have been imported; that is, the person became infected elsewhere but did not develop measles until after arrival from overseas.

Unfounded claims. Unfortunately, the extensive publicity given to the unfounded allegation that measles vaccine causes autism has made some parents afraid of the vaccine. Even though scientific studies have confirmed that there is no association between measles vaccine and autism, parents in some countries, such as England and Ireland, have refused to have their children vaccinated. And, as expected, when measles vaccination rates decrease, the number of cases of measles increases.

The Germ

How It Causes Illness

When droplets containing measles virus are breathed in, the virus first infects the cells lining the nose and throat. It then spreads to the lymph glands in the neck. After multiplying there for 2 to 3 days, the virus enters the blood and is carried throughout the body to other lymph glands, the liver, spleen and bone marrow where it grows for another

3 to 5 days. The virus then re-invades the blood and spreads to the skin, eyes, respiratory tract and other organs. The amount of virus in the blood reaches a peak about 11 to 14 days after exposure and then declines rapidly over a few days.

Two harmful proteins. The genes of the measles virus form an inner complex with three proteins, all of which is surrounded by a protective shell. Two proteins in the outer coat of the virus, called **hemagglutinin** (HA-protein) and the ***fusion protein*** (F-protein), play a very important role in creating infection.

The HA-protein attaches the virus to the cell. Then the F-protein fuses the virus coating to the outer membrane of the cell; this allows the genes of the virus to be transferred into the cell. Once inside, the viral genes take over the cell and make new viral particles. These infectious particles are reproduced and released. The "takeover" process (which starts with the HA-protein and the F-protein of the new viral particles) then repeats on other cells.

There is only **one known strain of measles virus.** However, minor differences in some of the genes and their proteins have been detected recently. It is not known whether these differences will alter the effectiveness of current measles vaccines, but they are cause for concern.

Damages many parts of the body. Measles, even without complications, causes damage to many parts of the body: the respiratory tract, lymph glands, spleen, liver, intestines and skin. Damage to the cells lining the nose and throat leads to a runny nose and sore throat. Damage to the bronchi (airways) results in a severe cough; almost all children with measles have bronchitis. As a result of multiplication of the virus in the lymph glands, liver and spleen, as well as inflammation, there is enlargement and often tenderness of these organs. Many infants and young children with measles get diarrhea as a result of damage to the intestinal tract.

Affects immune system. In addition to causing damage to many organs, measles also suppresses the major defences of the body against infection. Infection with measles virus affects the activity of the special cells of the immune system, called lymphocytes. Consequently, the ability of the immune system to respond to infection is markedly decreased for several months. Measles also lowers the activity of white blood cells responsible for killing bacteria.

Ear infections and pneumonia (an infection of the lungs) are common in children with measles because of the combination of damage to the lining of the respiratory tract and impaired defences against bacteria. The increased susceptibility to infection lasts several months after recovery from measles.

How Measles Virus Is Spread

Direct contact and airborne. Measles virus spreads very easily from person to person. An infected person may cough or sneeze, spreading droplets containing many virus particles. These particles may land in the nose or throat of another person, or become airborne (transported through the air). Measles virus is able to survive in small droplets in the air for at least several hours. This survival ability ensures airborne spread.

Highly contagious, easily spread. Airborne spread of measles virus explains the high level of contagiousness of the disease. Over 90% of susceptible persons exposed at home to a child with measles will catch it!

The type of illness brought on by the virus guarantees that the virus will spread. Most children have a runny nose, cough and fever for 2 to 4 days before the typical rash appears. During this time, large amounts of virus are present in the secretions in the nose, throat and bronchi. Therefore, the child is contagious before the illness is even diagnosed as measles. Children with measles are infectious to others for 8 days — 4 days before and 4 days after the start of the rash.

The Illness

Early symptoms (pre-rash). The incubation period for measles, or the time from exposure to the virus to the start of symptoms, is 10 to 12 days. The first symptoms are fever; aches and pains; runny nose; red, inflamed eyes; and cough. The fever increases over the first few days, usually reaching 39.4–40°C (103–104°F) by the time the rash appears. The cough is frequent and severe; bronchitis (infection of the airways) occurs in almost every case of measles.

These symptoms, similar to those of a bad cold, precede the start of the rash by 2 to 4 days. During this phase of the illness, spots may be seen in the mouth. These spots (called Koplik's spots) are unique to measles. They look like small grains of sand on a red base and are most often seen on the inner cheek opposite the molars. They disappear 1 to 2 days after the skin rash appears.

Rash. The rash consists of large red spots different from Koplik's spots. They appear first on the face and head, and spread down over the body to the arms and legs. The spots often become so large that there may be no normal skin in between, especially on the face and upper body. The rash begins to fade after about a week. The total illness lasts, on average, 7 to 14 days. The cough lasts longer than any of the other symptoms.

Complications

Complications are very common for two reasons: the infection causes extensive damage to the respiratory tract and impairs the function of white cells. Measles can cause death, even in previously healthy children. Complications and deaths are most common in infants (children less than 12 months old) and in adults. Even in the absence of complications, measles is a severe illness in children. Almost all children have high fever, severe cough, poor appetite, and are so sick that they are in bed for a week or more.

Rate of complications and related deaths. A complicating bacterial infection is likely present if the child's fever remains high for more than 2 days after onset of the rash, or if the child's fever recurs. Ear infections complicate measles in 7–9% of children, bacterial pneumonia occurs in 1–6%, and diarrhea in 6%. Approximately 1% of children are hospitalized because of measles or related complications. Death occurs in about 1 in every 1,000 cases. SSPE, a rare but fatal complication [see below], affects 1 in 100,000 measles patients.

The most common causes of death are pneumonia (an infection of the lungs) and encephalitis (an intense inflamation of the brain).

Pneumonia. Measles always infects the lower respiratory tract, causing bronchitis and cough. In 1–6% of cases, pneumonia develops, caused either by the measles virus itself or by secondary invasion of bacteria into areas damaged by measles. Pneumonia should be considered in any child who has a persistent or worsening cough and difficulty breathing. Treatment of pneumonia includes antibiotics, hospitalization, and oxygen if respiratory distress is severe.

Encephalitis occurs in about 1 in every 1,000 cases of measles. The symptoms of encephalitis include fever, seizures and marked impairment of consciousness. Many children go into coma. There is no effective treatment for measles encephalitis. About one-third of children with encephalitis die, one-third have significant brain damage and one-third recover. It can take a few weeks to many months to recover from encephalitis.

SSPE — rare but fatal. SSPE (subacute sclerosing panencephalitis) is a rare complication of measles, occurring in about 1 in every 100,000 cases. It is more common in children who have measles before age 2 than in those who have measles at an older age. SSPE is caused by chronic infection of brain cells with measles virus.

The illness begins about 7 years after the attack of measles. There is progressive destruction of nerve cells in the brain. As a result, patients with SSPE suffer from changes in personality and behaviour, loss of intellectual ability, seizures, and coma. There is no effective treatment, although some drugs have been shown to slow the rate of deterioration. SSPE is always fatal.

Measles during pregnancy. Infection of a pregnant woman with measles does not result in malformations of her baby. Measles, however, does cause a severe illness in adults, which does increase the risk of miscarriage and premature delivery.

Diagnosis

Any child with a red rash for 3 or more days, fever of 38.4°C (101°F) or higher, and cough, conjunctivitis (pink eye) and runny nose should be suspected of having measles. Because of the success of measles vaccination programs, most parents and physicians today have never seen a child with measles. Therefore, laboratory tests should be performed to confirm the diagnosis. The virus can be detected in saliva during the first few days of illness and specific antibody can be detected in the blood once the rash has started.

Treatment

No antibiotics. There is no specific treatment for measles. Antibiotics should not be prescribed in an attempt to prevent bacterial complications of measles. The rate of such complications is the same whether children are treated with antibiotics or not. There is a disadvantage to using antibiotics prematurely in the illness. If a child does develop complications, the bacteria involved in infection will more than likely have become resistant to the antibiotics because of prior treatment.

An **antiviral drug called ribavirin** is active against the measles virus and has been used to treat severely ill children. It is not yet clear how effective it is. Large doses of vitamin A have been shown to reduce the death rate from measles in infants and young children in developing countries. But children in many of these countries have inadequate intake of vitamin A due to poor nutrition. Such treatment is of little benefit in well-nourished children.

Immune globulin (IG) was used to prevent or modify measles before measles vaccine became available. IG is given by injection into muscle. It contains a large amount of antibody against measles virus. Antibodies coat the virus particles, enabling white blood cells to destroy the virus before it can cause any damage.

How is IG made? IG is prepared from plasma (the liquid part of blood) of blood donors using methods that concentrate the antibodies. When injected, the recipient gets a concentrated dose of measles antibody.

Is IG safe? Current methods of testing blood from volunteer donors and of preparing IG ensure that there is no risk of acquiring HIV, hepatitis B or hepatitis C from this product. Other than pain at the injection site, there are no significant reactions to IG.

Who should have IG?

Immune globulin (IG) is recommended for people who have been exposed to measles *and* who are at increased risk of severe disease and/or complications of measles, such as:
- infants (children less than 12 months old);
- pregnant women who have not had measles or measles vaccine;
- persons at risk because of problems with their immune system.

Does IG work? IG prevents measles in about 80% of exposed persons and reduces the severity of illness in most of those who do become ill. For IG to be effective, the injection must be given as soon as possible after exposure to measles. There is no benefit if more than 6 days have elapsed since exposure.

Post-recovery. Immunity following measles is lifelong.

The Vaccine

Type of Vaccine

Measles vaccine is a **live, attenuated vaccine**. This means that the vaccine is a live virus that multiplies in the body after it is given by injection. It is attenuated (weakened) compared with the wild strain, which causes "natural" measles. Even though it is able to multiply in the body after injection, it does not cause any illness in most people [see below, *Possible side effects of measles vaccine*].

How Measles Vaccine Is Made

Producing desirable strains. The measles virus was weakened by repeated infections of tissue culture cells. Each time the virus multiplies, mutations may occur in its genes, producing different strains of the virus. These strains are then tested in animals to determine if the virus has changed in the desired way. A "desirable" virus vaccine must be able to cause an infection but no longer cause damage. Once the desired strain has been isolated, large amounts of it are grown and stored for future production of vaccine.

Process. The weakened measles virus is grown in chick embryo cells. As the virus grows, it is released into the fluid covering the cells. An antibiotic, neomycin, is added to the culture fluid to prevent contamination with bacteria during production of the vaccine. The virus is extracted from the fluid, purified and sterilized. After passing all tests for potency (effectiveness) and safety [see below], the virus is freeze-dried, either alone or mixed with mumps and rubella vaccines. Before use, the freeze-dried (powdered form) vaccine must be mixed with sterile distilled water.

Additives. As stated above, neomycin is added to the culture fluid to prevent contamination with bacteria during production of the vaccine. Trace amounts (too small to be well defined) of this antibiotic remain in the vaccine. Sorbitol (sugar alcohol) and hydrolyzed (water-added) gelatin are added to stabilize the freeze-dried virus. The vaccine does *not* contain thimerosal, a mercury-containing preservative.

Testing. Tests for potency (effectiveness), toxicity and sterility are carried out on all batches of vaccine, both by the manufacturer and the Bureau of Biologics and Radiopharmaceuticals. [See Chapter 2.]

Available Forms of Measles Vaccine

The first measles vaccine was licensed in Canada and the United States in 1963. It was named the *Edmonston strain* after the child from whom the virus was isolated. By 1975, over 20 million doses had been given in the two countries!

A new strain in Canada since 1975. Because of the high occurrence rate of side effects (fever greater than 39.4°C [103°F] and rash) in children given the Edmonston strain of vaccine, researchers further attenuated the vaccine strains. The result: the new strains produce a much lower rate of fever and rash, yet are still effective in inducing a protective immune response. Several of these strains have been developed in different countries. The *Moraten strain* is used in Canada and the United States.

Combinations. In Canada, the combined measles, mumps and rubella (MMR) vaccine is used for routine vaccination of infants, given as a single injection. Measles vaccine is available on its own as well.

How the Vaccine Is Given

Beneath the skin. Measles vaccine is most often combined with mumps and rubella vaccines, producing a vaccine commonly known as MMR. The freeze-dried combination vaccine is supplied in a single vial; special preservative-free water is added just before it is used. The vaccine is given as a single injection beneath the skin (not into muscle).

Because exposure to sunlight or heat will kill the measles vaccine virus (even in the freeze-dried state), the vaccine must be refrigerated at the proper temperature (5–8°C/41–46°F). If the vaccine virus dies before it is injected, it will not be able to induce any protection.

Schedule of Vaccination

Infants and children (under age 7). In Canada and the United States, the routine immunization schedule consists of 2 doses of measles vaccine, given as the combined MMR vaccine. The first dose is given on or as soon after the first birthday as possible; the second dose is given at 4 to 6 years of age, before the child starts school. In a few Canadian provinces, the second dose is given at 18 months of age. Both schedules are effective.

Children (age 7 and over) and adults. All susceptible older children, adolescents and adults should be immunized. Persons should be considered to be susceptible to measles unless they have a written record of appropriate immunization, have immunity to measles documented by a laboratory test for measles antibody, or were born before 1957. (Because almost all adults born before 1957 were infected with measles, they do not need to be immunized.)

Boosters (to enhance prior vaccinations). Boosters are not required for anyone who has been properly immunized with 2 doses of MMR or MR vaccine.

Duration of protection. Immunity after 2 doses of measles vaccine lasts for many years, if not for life.

Possible Side Effects of Measles Vaccine

Mild. Side effects after measles vaccine, whether given alone or combined with mumps and rubella vaccines, are usually mild. Reactions occur only in those who are susceptible to measles. (Almost all children are susceptible at the time of the first dose; only a few have some remaining maternal antibody.) When children are given a second dose of measles vaccine, no reactions occur in those who are immune as a result of the first dose.

The illness caused by the vaccine (fever and rash) is much less severe and frequent [see below] than the illness associated with "natural" measles (fever, rash, cough and bronchitis lasting 7 to 14 days in 100% of cases).

Fever. The most common side effect of the vaccine is fever. It usually occurs 8 to 10 days after vaccination and lasts 24 to 48 hours. The fever may be high enough to cause a seizure in children who are susceptible to febrile seizures (those caused by fever). [For more detail on febrile convulsions, see Chapter 5, under *Possible side effects of pertussis vaccine*].

Rash due to the vaccine occurs in about 2% of children and also lasts 24 to 48 hours.

Studies of side effects in twins. The most detailed study of side effects after measles vaccination involved 580 twins in Finland. Half were given measles vaccine and the other half received an injection that didn't contain the vaccine (a placebo). One month later, every twin who had received the placebo injection was vaccinated, and those who had gotten the vaccine were given the placebo. Only the reactions that occurred more frequently after vaccine than after placebo could reasonably be attributed to vaccination.

The only symptom that occurred more frequently after measles vaccine than after placebo was fever. About 2% of the twins had fever of 39.4°C (103°F) or higher, occurring 8 to 10 days after vaccination.

Other studies. Most other studies of measles vaccine have found higher rates of side effects, with 5–15% of children having fever and rash. Unfortunately, these studies did not have a control group of unvaccinated children; so, many of the episodes of fever and rash blamed on the vaccine were probably due to other viral infections.

Severe adverse events rare. More severe adverse events after measles vaccine are very rare in healthy children. It is estimated that the risk of *encephalitis* after measles vaccine is less than 1 case per 1 million doses. Because this occurs so rarely, it is still not known whether the vaccine can cause encephalitis. Measles itself, on the other hand, causes encephalitis in about 1 of every 1,000 cases. In countries in which all children are vaccinated against measles, measles encephalitis has disappeared.

It is not known whether measles vaccine can cause **SSPE** [see *Complications*, above, for a description of SSPE]. As this illness has disappeared in countries with effective vaccination programs, such as Canada and the United States, it seems unlikely that the vaccine causes SSPE.

Study findings provide evidence that there is *no direct effect of measles vaccine on the brain*. EEG (electroencephalogram) tests were obtained on 40 children after measles vaccination. The EEG test measures the electrical activity of the brain. None of the vaccinated children had abnormal EEG tests. In contrast, one-half of children with uncomplicated measles (i.e., the natural illness) have abnormal EEGs.

Studies show no link to other diseases/disorders. Many studies have looked for other serious side effects of measles vaccine. However, there is no scientific evidence that measles vaccine (alone or combined in the MMR vaccine) causes autism or any other kind of brain damage or developmental delay. There is also no scientific proof that either measles vaccine or MMR vaccine causes Crohn's disease, ulcerative colitis or any other chronic inflammatory disease of the bowel. [See Chapter 17, Questions 22 and 24]. [For more information, see reports issued by the Institute of Medicine, at www.iom.edu/iom/iomhome.nsf/Pages/immunization+safety+review. See also Chapter 2.]

Increased susceptibility to infection after vaccination. Like wild measles virus, the vaccine strains also decrease the activity of the immune system for several months. However, the effect is much less pronounced after measles vaccination than after natural infection with measles. Increased susceptibility to infection has not been observed following measles vaccination of children who are 12 months of age or older.

Reasons to Avoid or Delay Measles Vaccine

Do not give. The National Advisory Committee on Immunization recognizes only one absolute reason not to give measles vaccine: an allergic reaction (hives; swelling of face, lips or throat; wheezing; or shock [fall in blood pressure]) to neomycin (an antibiotic that is in the vaccine), to gelatin, as to a previous dose of the measles vaccine.

Do not delay. In the past, it was recommended that *children who have allergic reactions after eating eggs* should not be vaccinated with measles or mumps vaccines, unless a special vaccine schedule was used. Because measles and mumps vaccines are grown in chick embryo cells, there has been concern that some of the proteins from the cells may be closely related to egg proteins. (Egg proteins are known to be the part of the egg that causes allergic reactions.)

Recent studies show that children with egg allergy can be safely vaccinated with measles and mumps vaccines without the need for special precautions. Most allergic reactions to MMR vaccine are now thought to be due to allergy to gelatin.

Vaccination should not be deferred or delayed because of *minor illnesses*, such as the common cold, with or without fever. Such infections do not increase the risk of side effects and do not interfere with the immune response to vaccination.

Measles vaccine is recommended and has been shown to be safe for *children infected with HIV or with AIDS who are not severely immunocompromised* (i.e., their immune systems are not severely impaired).

Delay. Vaccination should be delayed for the reasons indicated below.

Moderate to severe illness, with or without fever, is a reason to delay routine immunization. This precaution may be taken in order to avoid adding any side effects of the vaccine on top of the effects of the illness itself. However, if measles is occurring in the community, vaccination is recommended because the risk of measles in an unimmunized infant is much greater than the risk of any side effects.

Immunosuppression (lowered immune system). Measles is often very severe in persons with problems involving the immune system. (Problems result from underlying disease or medication.) Measles can be severe or fatal in persons with HIV infection. One would therefore assume that in these cases, the vaccine would be recommended. However, the original measles vaccine caused pneumonia in a few children with leukemia.

Therefore, it is recommended that measles vaccine *not* be given to persons with severe disorders of the immune system because of the risk of vaccine-related pneumonia. However, measles vaccine *is* recommended and has been shown to be safe for children infected with HIV or with AIDS who are not severely immunocompromised.

Pregnancy. Although measles does not infect the fetus or cause malformations, it is recommended that pregnant women not receive measles vaccine. However, children of a woman who is pregnant may be vaccinated; viruses contained in the measles, mumps and rubella vaccines do not spread from person to person.

Recent injection with IG or other blood products. Immune globulin (IG) and other blood products may contain antibody to measles virus that will interfere with the measles vaccine. Vaccination must be delayed for 3 to 11 months, depending on the type and dose of IG or other blood product used.

The Results of Vaccination

Vaccine strain doesn't spread. The immune response following measles vaccine is very similar to that after infection with wild measles virus. Although the vaccine virus does multiply in the body, it has never been detected in the blood following vaccination and is not excreted from the nose or throat. Therefore, the vaccine strain does not spread from a vaccinated child to another person.

Long-lasting protection. Protective antibodies appear in the blood within 12 days of vaccination and reach peak concentrations within 21 to 28 days. The amount of antibody induced by the vaccine is lower than that observed after measles. Nevertheless, immunity persists for many years after vaccination.

When measles vaccine is given in combination with mumps and rubella vaccines, the same immune responses are observed as when each vaccine is given separately. The combined MMR vaccine can also be given at the same time as any of the following vaccines without affecting the immune responses to the vaccines or the rates of side effects:

- DTaP (diphtheria and tetanus toxoids, and acellular pertussis) vaccine;
- IPV or OPV (inactivated polio vaccine or oral polio) vaccine;
- Hib (*Haemophilus influenzae* type b) vaccine;
- chickenpox (varicella) vaccine.

Vaccine Failure — Reasons

Maternal antibody. About 5–10% of infants fail to respond to the first dose of measles vaccine. A number of reasons have been found to explain such failures. The most important reason is antibody against measles that is transferred from a mother to her baby near the end of pregnancy. If the quantity of maternal antibodies transferred to the baby is great enough, the live virus the child receives by vaccine will be destroyed before it can stimulate the baby's immune system.

Antibodies received from the mother disappear over time. By their first birthday, 9 out of 10 babies have lost the maternal antibody and can be successfully vaccinated.

Mothers whose immunity to measles is the result of vaccination have lower amounts of antibody than mothers who had measles in childhood. An increasing proportion of mothers today had vaccine, not measles. Therefore, more and more babies will have less measles antibody from their mothers. This should result in a decrease of the frequency of vaccine failures after the first dose.

Vaccine storage. Improper storage of measles vaccine is the second most important cause of vaccine failure. Exposure to sunlight or heat will kill the vaccine virus. Because the vaccine virus must be alive when it is injected, the vaccine must be stored at 5–8°C (41–46°F) at all times (even when freeze-dried) until it is used.

Previous one-dose immunization schedule. Because measles vaccine is not 100% effective and because not all children are vaccinated, measles continued to occur in Canada long after the start of routine vaccination (in 1963). Many cases occurred in vaccinated children, especially in outbreaks in schools. Why?

Each dose of measles vaccine is about 95% effective when administered on or after the first birthday. For example, if all 100 children in a school are vaccinated, 5 will still be susceptible after 1 dose. If a case occurs in this school where only 5 of 100 children are susceptible, measles is so highly contagious that the infection will most likely spread to all 5 children — even though they have received 1 dose of vaccine.

Vaccine Failure — Remedies

Two-dose schedule. Because of the problem of vaccine failure, many countries have adopted a two-dose schedule whereby children are given 1 dose of measles vaccine in infancy and a second before starting school. The purpose of the second dose is to ensure that the number of children who remain susceptible is less than 5%.

For example, in the school described above, 5 of the 100 children had not been protected by 1 dose of measles vaccine. If all 100 children were given a second dose of vaccine before starting school, at least 4 of the 5 susceptible children would be vaccinated successfully by the second dose. Measles would not be able to spread in that school because at least 99 of 100 children would be immune.

Studies of outbreaks in schools in Ontario confirm this theory: no cases occurred in children who had received 2 or more doses of measles vaccine.

Vaccine Success

Evidence that measles vaccine works includes the following:

Mass campaigns. Because of the persistence of measles outbreaks in school children, all Canadian provinces and territories have adopted a two-dose measles vaccination schedule. A mass vaccination program was undertaken in Ontario and Quebec in the spring of 1996. All children attending school were vaccinated to prevent additional school outbreaks. Such mass campaigns have been shown to be very effective in interrupting the spread of measles among school-age children in the United Kingdom, Cuba and English-speaking islands of the Caribbean.

Lifelong immunity. A group of 70 children were all found to have measles antibody 16 years after receiving just 1 dose of measles vaccine. A larger study involving 1,871 high school students found that 98.8% had measles antibody 14 to 16 years after receiving 1 dose of vaccine. Immunity after 2 doses is expected to be lifelong.

Proposals to eradicate measles. Measles vaccination programs have been successful in greatly reducing the frequency of measles.

They have been so successful, in fact, that **global eradication** of measles has been proposed by the World Health Organization. But worldwide eradication of measles will prove to be more difficult than that of polio and smallpox. Eradication in Third World countries will be especially difficult for the following reasons:

- In most underdeveloped countries, the high rate of population growth means that increasing numbers of susceptible children are living under conditions that facilitate the spread of measles, namely overcrowding, poverty and lack of effective health care.
- Measles vaccine is not 100% effective, and the infection is highly contagious.
- Measles vaccine must be kept refrigerated at the proper temperature.

Canada has accepted measles eradication as a **national immunization goal**. To achieve eradication in Canada, all children must receive their first dose of vaccine by 15 months of age and their second dose before they enter school.

Summary

- Measles is not "an ordinary infection that all children should have."
- Having measles is of no benefit to a child (except that it provides immunity to the infection).
- Measles was, and is, a severe illness with a high rate of complications and a real risk of permanent disability and death.
- Measles vaccine provides the same protection against measles that the natural illness provides — without the risk of severe illness or complications.
- All children should be vaccinated against measles.
- Measles vaccine is very safe.
- Measles vaccine does not cause autism, Crohn's disease or other forms of bowel disease.

- Two doses of measles vaccine are necessary because about 5% of vaccinated children remain unprotected following the first dose.
- There are some obstacles to overcome in order for global measles vaccination programs to be completely successful; with perseverance and time, it will be possible to eradicate measles.

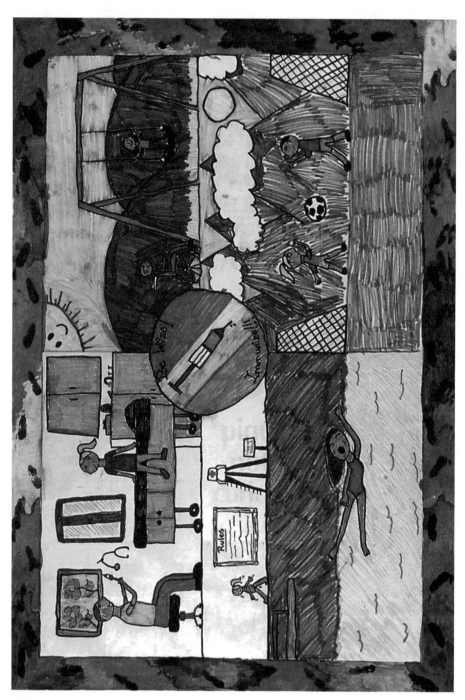

Miranda Angel, Haines Junction, Yukon Territory

CHAPTER 9

Mumps

Mumps is an infection caused by the mumps virus. This infection can cause fever, headache, and swelling of the salivary glands around the jaw and cheeks. Mumps can also cause meningitis, an infection of the fluid and lining that cover the brain and spinal cord. About 1 in every 10 people with mumps gets meningitis. Mumps meningitis is usually mild and does not cause permanent damage.

Mumps can also cause encephalitis (intense inflammation of the brain), which may lead to permanent brain damage. Other complications of mumps include deafness, painful swelling of the testicles in teenage boys and men, and painful infection of the ovaries in women. In rare cases, men with both testicles infected with mumps become sterile.

The second "M" in MMR vaccine stands for mumps.

A History of Mumps

Before Vaccine

Before the introduction of mumps vaccine, about 30,000 cases of mumps were reported annually in Canada. This number was much lower than the actual number for two reasons: physicians did not always report cases and, more importantly, many cases of mumps were so mild that the patients were not seen by a physician.

In 1980–81, a detailed study of mumps was carried out in Alberta. During this one-year period, 1 out of every 6 susceptible children was infected with mumps. The study showed that the number and severity of complications of mumps were not great enough to be considered a major problem. Mumps was usually a mild disease.

Nevertheless, when the safety, effectiveness and cost of mumps vaccine were compared with the costs of treating patients with mumps, it was clear that immunization would benefit children and save money. Savings would be greatest if the vaccine could be combined with measles and rubella vaccines.

After Vaccine

Data from Canada, the United States, France, the United Kingdom, Sweden and Finland show that the number of cases of mumps decreased by over 90% after mumps vaccine became available.

Before mumps vaccination programs began in the early 1970s, mumps was the most common cause of encephalitis (inflamation of the brain) in children. Mumps encephalitis has virtually disappeared from countries with effective vaccination programs. The average annual number of cases reported between 1998 and 2000 in Canada following the implementation of the two-dose MMR vaccination schedule throughout Canada was 95, a 99.7% decline from the number of reported cases prior to the introduction of mumps vaccine.

The Germ

How It Causes Illness

Mumps is a viral infection, and it starts as an infection of the nose and throat. The virus spreads through the blood to many parts of the body. The most common feature in those with mumps is painful swelling of the salivary glands. As a result of spread of the virus through the blood, other body parts that may be infected include the covering of the brain and spinal cord, testicles or ovaries, pancreas, kidneys, breasts, thyroid, joints and inner ears.

How Mumps Is Spread

Direct contact. Spread of mumps virus requires close, direct contact between people. An infected person may cough or sneeze, spreading droplets containing many virus particles. These particles may land in the nose or throat of another person. Indirect spread of mumps virus through the air or on contaminated toys or other objects does not occur very often.

Duration of contagious period. Children with mumps are contagious from about 2 days before the start of swelling of the salivary glands until up to 9 days after the start of swelling. The many children (almost 60%) infected with mumps who do not develop swollen glands or other significant symptoms can also spread the virus.

The Illness

Nine out of 10 infections with mumps virus occur in children under the age of 15. More than half of those children are 5 to 9 years of age. The frequency of mumps is the same in boys and girls.

Symptoms. The incubation period of mumps (time from exposure to onset of symptoms) is longer than that of measles or chickenpox. Illness develops an average of 16 to 18 days after exposure. About 20% of children infected with mumps virus have no symptoms at all; 40% have a minor illness similar to a cold; and 40% get swollen salivary glands (typical mumps, as described below).

Adults and children less than 2 years of age are more likely than preschool and young school-age children to have mild infections without salivary gland involvement.

Typical illness. Mumps usually starts with fever, aches and pains, and loss of appetite. Other symptoms in children with mumps include headache in 40%; neck stiffness in 33%; stomach ache in 20%; and drowsiness, confusion or dizziness in 15%.

After 1 or more days, the salivary glands become swollen and painful. The parotid gland (the largest of the salivary glands, located in front of the ear behind the angle of the jaw) is affected in 90% of those with swollen glands. Both sides are enlarged in about half of cases; there are an equal number of single-left and single-right cases. Other salivary glands are affected in 30–40% of cases.

Duration of illness. When mumps was a common illness, the average duration of illness was as follows: fever lasted 3 days; pain, 5 days; swelling, 8 days; and confinement to bed, 3 days. The number of days off work or out of school was 7. Parents stayed home for an average of 1 day to care for the child. Most children were back to normal within 14 days.

Mumps is less contagious than measles or chickenpox. Studies show that only one-third of susceptible family members get mumps following an illness in a child.

Complications

Meningitis is the most common complication of mumps. It is caused by direct invasion of the membranes and fluid covering the brain and spinal cord by mumps virus. Most cases are very mild and symptoms such as headache, neck stiffness and drowsiness last only a few days. The illness is rarely severe and almost never causes permanent damage. It occurs in approximately 5% (1 out of 20) of cases of mumps.

Mumps encephalitis (inflammation of the brain) is caused by an allergic reaction of the body to mumps infection. Mumps encephalitis occurs more frequently in adults than in children. Permanent brain damage may occur and lead to problems such as recurrent seizures, paralysis or hydrocephalus (excess fluid on the brain).

Infection with mumps virus can cause **deafness** in children. Deafness is caused by damage to the auditory nerve and/or inner ear. It is estimated to occur in 1 out of every 200,000 cases. Deafness may occur without any other signs of involvement of the brain, such as meningitis or encephalitis.

In males. Mumps infection of the testicles (orchitis) is rare before puberty. However, about 20–40% of men with mumps get orchitis. Most cases involve only one testicle and recovery is complete. Sterility after mumps orchitis is rare, even when both testicles are infected.

In females. Adult women with mumps may get painful swelling of the breasts and abdominal or pelvic pain due to inflammation of the ovaries. There is no proof that mumps causes infertility.

During pregnancy. There is no risk of malformations of the fetus if a woman is infected with mumps while she is pregnant. As with any infection during pregnancy, a severe illness can result in miscarriage.

Mumps infection causes **inflammation of the pancreas** (pancreatitis) in about 4% of cases, with vomiting and abdominal pain. An association between mumps pancreatitis and diabetes has been suggested, but has not been proven.

Diagnosis

Clinical examination. The diagnosis of mumps is usually made on the basis of the typical painful swelling of the parotid glands (largest salivary glands). However, other viruses (such as influenza, parainfluenza and adenovirus) can cause an illness identical to mumps. Up to one-third of cases of acute swelling of the parotid glands are not caused by mumps.

Laboratory tests. The diagnosis can be confirmed by finding mumps virus in saliva, urine or other body fluids during the first 5 days after onset of illness. Tests to detect increases in the amount of mumps antibody in the blood can also be used to make the diagnosis.

Treatment

For symptoms only. There is no effective treatment for mumps. Pain can be reduced with acetaminophen (e.g., Tempra, Tylenol). Hot or cold compresses may also ease the pain in the salivary glands.

Post-recovery. Although it is possible to be infected with mumps more than once, such events are rare. Most recurrent cases of "mumps" turn out to be illnesses caused by other viruses. Persons infected with mumps virus develop lifelong immunity whether the glands were swollen or not.

The Vaccine

Type of Vaccine

Live, attenuated virus. Mumps vaccine is a live virus vaccine that has been attenuated (weakened). This means that the vaccine contains a live virus that multiplies in the body after it is given by injection. It is attenuated compared with the wild strain, which causes natural mumps infection. The vaccine virus does not cause any illness in most people [see below, *Possible side effects of mumps vaccine*]. It does, however, mimic natural infection: the virus infects, multiplies and stimulates immunity.

How Mumps Vaccine Is Made

Producing desirable strains. The mumps virus was attenuated or weakened by repeated growth in hens' eggs, and then in chick embryo cell cultures. Each time the virus multiplies, mutations may occur in its genes, producing different strains of the virus. These strains are then tested to determine if the virus has changed in the desired way. A "desirable" virus vaccine must be able to cause an infection but no longer cause damage. Once the desired strain has been isolated, large amounts of it are grown and stored for future production of vaccine.

The vaccine strain used in Canada and the United States is called the *Jeryl Lynn strain,* after the child from whom it was isolated. Nine other vaccine strains have been developed and are used in other countries.

Process. The Jeryl Lynn strain of mumps vaccine virus is grown in chick embryo cells. As the virus grows, it is released into the fluid covering the cells. An antibiotic, neomycin, is added to the culture fluid to prevent contamination with bacteria during production of the vaccine. The virus is extracted from the fluid, purified and sterilized. After passing all tests for potency and safety, the virus is freeze-dried, either alone or mixed with measles and rubella vaccines. Before use, the powdered vaccine must be mixed with sterile distilled water.

Additives. As stated above, neomycin is added to the culture fluid to prevent contamination with bacteria during production of the vaccine. Trace amounts (too small to be well defined) of this antibiotic remain in the vaccine. Sorbitol (sugar alcohol) and hydrolyzed (water-added) gelatin are added to stabilize the freeze-dried virus. The vaccine does *not* contain thimerosal, a mercury-containing preservative.

Testing. Tests for potency (effectiveness), toxicity and sterility are carried out on all batches of vaccine, by both the manufacturer and the Bureau of Biologics and Radiopharmaceuticals. [See *Vaccine safety* in Chapter 2 for more detail.]

Available Forms of Mumps Vaccine

Combinations. In Canada, the combined measles, mumps and rubella (MMR) vaccine is used for routine vaccination of infants, given as a single injection. Mumps vaccine is also available by itself.

Vaccines for older children and adults. The same dosage of vaccine is used for everyone.

How the Vaccine Is Given

The freeze-dried combination MMR vaccine is mixed with distilled water and given as a single injection beneath the skin (into the tissues overlying the muscle).

Exposure to sunlight or heat will kill mumps vaccine virus. The vaccine must be refrigerated at the proper temperature (5–8°C/41–46°F). If the vaccine virus dies before it is injected, it won't be able to stimulate the immune responses. Improper storage remains a problem and may be responsible for failures of the vaccine.

Schedule of Vaccination

Infants and children (under age 7). In Canada and the United States, the routine immunization schedule consists of 2 doses of mumps vaccine, given as the combined MMR vaccine. The first dose is given on or as soon after the first birthday as possible; the second dose is given at 4 to 6 years of age, before the child starts school. In a few Canadian provinces, the second dose is given at 18 months of age. Both schedules are effective.

Children (age 7 and over) and adults. Two doses of MMR (or mumps vaccine on its own) are given at least 1 month apart.

Boosters (to enhance prior vaccinations). Boosters are not required if 2 doses of MMR have been given.

Duration of protection. After 2 doses of vaccine, protection lasts many years, if not for life.

Possible Side Effects of Mumps Vaccine

Rare with Jeryl Lynn strain. Side effects of the Jeryl Lynn strain of mumps vaccine have been rare. A few children develop swelling of the salivary glands 10 to 14 days after vaccination. Meningitis has been reported to occur at a rate of 1 case per 800,000 doses.

Comparison with another vaccine strain. A different mumps vaccine, called the *Urabe vaccine strain*, causes meningitis much more frequently than the Jeryl Lynn vaccine. Studies in Canada, Japan, France and the United Kingdom have found that the rate of meningitis after injection of the Urabe vaccine is 1 case per 60,000 doses.

Because the occurrence rate is more than 10 times higher with this strain than with the Jeryl Lynn strain, the Urabe strain is no longer approved for use in Canada or the United States. Even though the rate of 1 case in 60,000 doses is high (compared with 1 in 800,000 with the Jeryl Lynn strain), it is still much lower than the risk of meningitis with natural mumps infection [see Table below].

TABLE 9.1

Occurrence rate of mumps meningitis, by source of virus

SOURCE OF MUMPS VIRUS	FREQUENCY OF MENINGITIS
Natural infection	1 in 20 cases
Vaccine – Urabe strain	1 in 60,000 doses
Vaccine – Jeryl Lynn strain	1 in 800,000 doses

No permanent brain damage has occurred after the rare cases of meningitis or encephalitis (inflammation of the brain) caused by mumps vaccine.

Reasons to Avoid or Delay Mumps Vaccine

Do not give. The National Advisory Committee on Immunization recognizes only one absolute reason not to give mumps vaccine: an allergic reaction (hives; swelling of face, lips or throat; wheezing; or shock [fall in blood pressure]) to neomycin (an antibiotic that is in the vaccine), to gelatin, or to a previous dose of mumps vaccine.

Do not delay. In the past, it was recommended that *children who have allergic reactions after eating eggs* should not be vaccinated with measles or mumps vaccines, unless a special vaccine schedule was used. Because measles and mumps vaccines are grown in chick embryo cells, there has been concern that some of the proteins from the cells may be closely related to egg proteins. (Egg proteins are known to be the part of the egg that causes allergic reactions.) Recent studies show that children with egg allergy can be safely vaccinated with measles and mumps vaccines without the need for special precautions. Most allergic reactions to MMR vaccine are now thought to be due to allergy to gelatin.

Vaccination should not be deferred or delayed because of **minor illnesses**, such as the common cold, with or without fever. Such infections do not increase the risk of side effects and do not interfere with the immune response to vaccination.

Mumps vaccine is recommended and has been shown to be safe for **children infected with HIV or AIDS who are not severely immunocompromised**.

Delay. Vaccination should be delayed for the reasons indicated below.

Moderate to severe illness, with or without fever, is a reason to delay routine immunization. This precaution may be taken in order to avoid adding any side effects of the vaccine on top of the effects of the illness itself.

Immunosuppression (lowered immune system). Mumps vaccine, as with all live virus vaccines, should not be given to persons with serious disorders of the immune system caused by underlying disease or medication.

Pregnancy. Although mumps does not infect the fetus or cause malformations, the safety of this vaccine during pregnancy has not yet been proven. Therefore, it is recommended that pregnant women not receive mumps vaccine. However, children of a woman who is pregnant may be vaccinated; the virus contained in the mumps vaccine does not spread from person to person.

Recent injection with IG or other blood products. Immune globulin (IG) and other blood products may contain antibody to mumps virus that will interfere with the mumps vaccine. Vaccination must be delayed for 3 to 11 months, depending on the type and dose of IG or other blood product used.

The Results of Vaccination

Over 90% of those vaccinated are protected against mumps. The vaccine provides the same protection whether given separately or combined with measles and rubella vaccines.

Evidence that mumps vaccine works includes the following:
- Controlled studies demonstrated that a single dose of mumps vaccine is over 90% effective in preventing mumps.
- The average annual number of cases reported between 1998 and 2000 in Canada following the implementation of the two-dose MMR vaccination schedule throughout Canada was 95, a 99.7% decline from the number of reported cases prior to the introduction of mumps vaccine.

Because the amount of antibody induced by the vaccine is considerably less than that induced by natural infection, there has been concern about the duration of protection after vaccination. Small outbreaks of mumps still occur, mainly in vaccinated teenagers and young adults (ages 13 to 25). It has not been determined whether this vaccine failure is due to lack of response to the vaccine or to gradual loss of immunity. Introduction of a routine two-dose schedule of MMR vaccination has reduced the occurrence of such outbreaks.

Summary

- Mumps is a relatively mild infection without a high risk of severe complications. However, it can cause permanent brain damage and deafness.
- Mumps vaccine is very safe and effective.
- The ability to combine mumps vaccine with measles and rubella vaccines into a single product (MMR) makes mumps vaccine very cost-effective. In addition, the costs of doctor visits for mumps infection are eliminated, as are costs associated with parents staying home from work to care for children sick with the mumps.
- All children should be vaccinated against mumps.

Education and Immunization

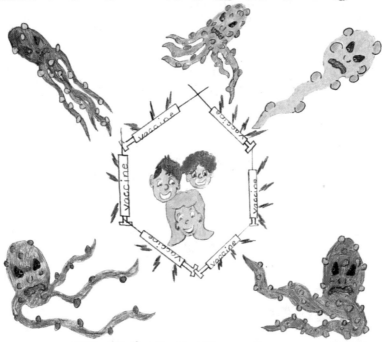

POWERFUL
DEFENCE
against infection

Andrew Merrithew, Miramichi, New Brunswick

CHAPTER 10

Rubella

Rubella, also known as German measles, is an infection caused by a virus. Rubella can lead to fever, sore throat, swollen glands, and small red spots that last a few days. Rubella is usually a mild illness in children. Many children don't even get a fever or rash, and sometimes the infection causes no symptoms at all. Rubella is usually more severe in teenagers and adults.

The most serious problem caused by rubella occurs if a woman is infected during the first 20 weeks of pregnancy. The virus can infect the fetus and cause malformations of the brain, eyes, ears, heart and other organs, and even death. This is called congenital rubella syndrome. Most children born with this syndrome are severely handicapped.

The "R" in MMR vaccine stands for rubella.

A History of Rubella

Before Vaccine

Women at risk. In North America, outbreaks of rubella occurred almost every spring, mainly in children aged 6 to 10. Larger epidemics occurred about every 7 years. Approximately 85% of people had had rubella by the time they reached 20 years of age. (This means that approximately 250,000 rubella infections occurred every year in Canada prior to the introduction of rubella vaccine.) The remaining 15% of people were therefore still susceptible to rubella. At greatest risk in this group were the women of child-bearing age, who were at risk of becoming infected while pregnant.

An eye doctor in Australia first noted the *danger of rubella during pregnancy* in 1941. Dr. Alan Gregg cared for a number of infants who had been born with cataracts. He discovered that the mothers of these infants had rubella during the early part of their pregnancies. Other doctors in many other parts of the world confirmed his findings. It was also found that many of the infants were deaf and had malformed hearts.

Epidemic in 1964. Rubella virus was first isolated and grown in a laboratory in 1962, shortly before a worldwide epidemic of rubella began in 1964. During this epidemic, it is estimated that about 12.5 million cases of rubella occurred in the United States alone. Nearly 30,000 babies were infected with rubella during the first 20 weeks of pregnancy. Of these babies, more than 8,000 died and about 20,000 had congenital rubella syndrome.

This epidemic was extraordinary in size. For comparison, in an "average" year (non-epidemic conditions) in the United States, about 2,000 babies would be born with congenital rubella syndrome.

After Vaccine

Three different rubella vaccines were developed and licensed in 1968–69. The goal of rubella vaccination programs was — and still is — to prevent congenital rubella syndrome. At first, the vaccine was used in two different ways in different countries.

American strategy. The United States and several Canadian provinces used a three-step program:
1. All children should be vaccinated at about 1 year of age.
2. All women of child-bearing age should be tested for immunity to rubella.
3. Women with negative results should be vaccinated.

The American strategy was designed to stop the spread of rubella by vaccinating all children. Stopping the spread of rubella would prevent susceptible pregnant women from being exposed to the virus.

British plan. In other Canadian provinces and the United Kingdom, the vaccine was recommended only for girls 10 to 12 years of age and susceptible adult women. The theory behind this so-called British plan was that the combined effects of rubella infection of young boys and girls and vaccination of 10- to 12-year-old girls would eventually lead to fewer women being susceptible to rubella. However, only about 85% of schoolgirls actually received the rubella vaccine, so the plan was not as effective as had been hoped.

A clear winner. The occurrence rate of congenital rubella syndrome in the United Kingdom and in Canadian provinces using the British plan did not fall as much or as rapidly as in the United States and provinces using the American strategy. In 1983, a review of the British plan led to the adoption by all Canadian provinces and territories of the American strategy of rubella vaccination of all infants.

In October 1988, British authorities changed to the American schedule. After that date, rubella vaccination, given as the combined measles, mumps and rubella vaccine (MMR), was recommended for all infants in the United Kingdom.

Today, success. No major epidemics have occurred since 1965. Since the start of routine rubella vaccination (in 1980), the number of babies born in Canada with congenital rubella syndrome has declined from approximately 200 per year to an average of 3, a decline of 98.5%. All of the cases have occurred in babies whose mothers had never had either the disease or the vaccine before becoming infected while pregnant.

The Germ

How It Causes Illness

After droplets containing rubella virus are breathed in, the virus first infects the cells lining the nose and throat. It then spreads to the lymph glands in the neck. After about 2 weeks, the virus then invades the blood and spreads to the skin, eyes, respiratory tract and other organs. Onset of the rash indicates the peak of infection and the beginning of recovery.

During pregnancy. While rubella virus is in the blood of a pregnant woman, it can infect the placenta and then the fetus. Rubella infection of the fetus (in the womb) differs from infection of a baby (after birth). Cells of the embryo and developing fetus are unable to get rid of the virus. Infection of the fetal cells prevents normal cell division. Normal growth and development of many organs is interrupted, resulting in the typical malformations of babies with congenital rubella syndrome.

How Rubella Is Spread

Direct contact. Spread of rubella virus requires close, direct contact between people. An infected person may cough or sneeze, spreading droplets containing many virus particles. These droplets may land in the nose or throat of another person. The virus is present in the throat of the infected person from about 7 days before the start of the rash to 2 weeks after.

Duration of contagious period. Contagiousness is at its peak a few days before the rash appears and declines rapidly thereafter. Rubella virus is excreted for more than a year by babies born with congenital rubella syndrome. Consequently, these babies are contagious for a year or more after birth because rubella virus is in the saliva and urine, and can easily be spread.

Less contagious than other illnesses. Rubella is not as contagious as other childhood infections, such as measles or chickenpox. In the era before vaccination, about 85% of children got rubella compared with over 95% who caught measles and chickenpox.

The Illness

Symptoms. The incubation period of rubella (time from exposure to the virus to start of symptoms) is 14 to 21 days. During the first week after exposure to rubella, no symptoms occur. During the second week, lymph glands may enlarge, especially behind the ears and at the back of the head.

At the end of the second week, a mild illness may begin with low-grade fever, aches and pains, and redness of the eyes. The characteristic rash [described below] usually appears after 1 or 2 days of mild illness. If the lymph glands did not enlarge earlier, they would most likely do so with the start of other symptoms.

Rash. The rash consists of small red spots, which appear first on the face and scalp. The rash spreads rapidly down the body and begins to fade within 1 to 3 days. The rubella rash is very similar to rashes caused by many other viral infections, making it difficult to diagnose rubella from the rash alone.

Rubella is usually much **milder in young children** than in adolescents and adults. Many children have either no illness at all or a mild illness without any rash. Adolescents and adults are much more likely to have symptoms and complications.

Complications

Joint pain. The most common complication of rubella is pain in the joints. Involvement of the joints occurs more frequently in adults (especially women) than in children. It is not known why women are much more likely than men to have joint pain from rubella. Most women who experience joint pain after rubella infection do not have actual arthritis (i.e., there is no redness, swelling or limitation of movement). The joint symptoms last a few days to a few weeks and almost always clear completely.

Rarely, chronic arthritis may develop after rubella. It is not clear whether rubella virus causes the arthritis, triggers an underlying joint disease, or is completely unrelated to the subsequent chronic joint problems.

Other complications of rubella infection are uncommon. A few children develop a condition called **thrombocytopenia**, characterized by a temporary decrease in the number of platelets (particles in the blood responsible for blood clot formation). Because of this decrease, small hemorrhages and bruises can occur in the skin. Although rare, major problems can result from this condition, especially if there is bleeding into the brain. The platelet problem goes away when infection resolves.

Encephalitis (inflammation of the brain) occurs in about 1 in 6,000 cases of rubella. It is more common in adults than in children. Encephalitis in rubella cases is the result of an allergic-type reaction of the body to the presence of the virus. The virus does *not* invade the brain cells as it does in most other types of encephalitis. Symptoms disappear over time and permanent brain damage is uncommon after rubella.

SSPE. Rubella can cause another, very different kind of encephalitis, called SSPE (subacute sclerosing panencephalitis). Most cases of SSPE are caused by measles, but it can also occur after rubella. Most cases have occurred in children with congenital rubella syndrome. SSPE is caused by persistent infection of brain cells with rubella virus. The illness begins years after the actual rubella infection.

SSPE caused by rubella is no different than SSPE caused by measles. Progressive destruction of nerve cells in the brain occurs as the immune system attacks the infected cells. As a result, children suffer progressive deterioration: changes in personality and behaviour; loss of intellectual ability; seizures; and coma. There is no treatment for SSPE, although some drugs may slow the rate of deterioration. The disease is always fatal.

Congenital rubella syndrome. When a pregnant woman is infected with rubella sometime during the first 20 weeks of pregnancy, chances are high (more than 8 in 10) that the fetus will also be infected. If the mother is infected *before* conception, rubella virus does not infect the fetus.

The stage of pregnancy during which the woman becomes infected determines the degree of damage suffered by the fetus. If infection occurs in the first 12 weeks of pregnancy, the baby is usually born with multiple handicaps [see Table 10.1, below]; if infection occurs between 16 and 20 weeks, deafness is usually the only complication. Infection after 20 weeks of pregnancy does not affect the fetus.

A fetus infected with rubella virus almost always sustains damage. In about 1 of 5 fetal infections, the damage is so severe that the fetus dies and the woman has a miscarriage. One of every 10 infected babies dies of complications in the first 12 months of life.

Infection causes two types of abnormalities:
• infection of fetal cells interferes with cell division so that organs may be malformed, such as the brain, heart, eyes and ears;
• other organs are affected because the virus kills cells directly, causing inflammation, as in the liver, spleen and bone marrow.

TABLE 10.1

Malformations associated with congenital rubella syndrome

BODY PART AFFECTED	RESULTING ABNORMALITY
General body	Low birth weight, impaired growth
Brain	Abnormally small brain, mental retardation, autism, SSPE
Eye	Cataracts, absent or small eyes, glaucoma, blindness
Ear	Deafness
Heart	Malformation
Liver	Hepatitis
Bone marrow	Low platelet count causing bleeding
Lung	Chronic pneumonia
Pancreas	Diabetes
Thyroid	Hypothyroidism

Diagnosis

Blood test. Many viral infections can cause an illness identical to rubella, right down to the same rash. Accurate diagnosis of rubella, therefore, requires a blood test to detect elevations in antibody to rubella. This is the same test used to detect antibody in women before or during pregnancy. [For more information on antibody and pregnancy, see *Schedule of vaccination*, below.]

Treatment

There is no treatment for rubella. Symptoms (such as headache, aches and pains, and joint pain) can be relieved with acetaminophen (e.g., Tylenol, Tempra). The damage associated with congenital rubella syndrome is irreversible.

The Vaccine

Type of Vaccine

Rubella vaccine is a **live, attenuated vaccine**. This means that the vaccine contains a live virus that multiplies in the body after it is given by injection. Attenuated means that it is weakened, compared with the wild strain that causes natural infection with rubella. The vaccine virus does not cause any illness in most people [see below, *Possible side effects of rubella vaccine*]. It does, however, mimic natural infection: the virus infects, multiplies and stimulates immunity.

How Rubella Vaccine Is Made

Producing desirable strains. A number of different rubella vaccines were developed in the late 1960s. The vaccine currently used in Canada, the United States, and all other countries except Japan is called **the RA27/3 vaccine**. The virus in the RA27/3 vaccine was isolated, then weakened in human embryonic cells called **WI-38 cells**.

About the WI-38 cells. These cells were derived from a single aborted fetus many decades ago and have been studied for a long time. They are free of any other viruses. All of the WI-38 cells used to produce vaccine were derived from this single fetus. The cells were grown in tissue culture; then samples of them were frozen and saved for future use. Production of the RA27/3 vaccine does *not* require cells from additional aborted fetuses.

Weakening the strain. The RA27/3 vaccine strain was attenuated by repeatedly growing it in the WI-38 tissue culture cells. Use of human cells to grow the vaccine reduces the risk of allergic reactions. Each time the virus multiplies, mutations may occur in its genes, producing different strains of the virus.

These strains are then tested in animals to determine if the virus has weakened in the desired way. A "desirable" virus must be able to cause infection but no longer causes illness or damage. Once a desirable strain has been isolated, large amounts of it are grown and stored for future production of vaccine.

Process. As the virus grows, it is released into the fluid covering the cells. An antibiotic, neomycin, is added to the culture fluid to prevent contamination with bacteria during production of the vaccine. The virus is extracted from the fluid, purified and sterilized. After passing all tests for potency (effectiveness) and safety [see below], the virus is freeze-dried, either alone or mixed with measles and mumps vaccines. Before use, the powdered vaccine must be mixed with sterile distilled water.

Additives. As stated above, neomycin is added to the culture fluid to prevent contamination with bacteria during production of the vaccine. Trace amounts (too small to be well defined) of this antibiotic remain in the vaccine. Sorbitol (sugar alcohol) and hydrolyzed (water-added) gelatin are added to stabilize the freeze-dried virus. The vaccine does *not* contain thimerosal, a mercury-containing preservative.

Testing. Tests for potency, toxicity and sterility are carried out on all batches of vaccine, by both the manufacturer and the Bureau of Biologics and Radiopharmaceuticals [see Chapter 2].

Available Forms of Rubella Vaccine

Combinations. In Canada, the combined measles, mumps and rubella (MMR) vaccine is used for routine vaccination of infants, given as a single injection. Rubella vaccine is also available in Canada in a combined measles–rubella (MR) vaccine.

Rubella vaccine is not provided on its own because of the low demand for it. Women who don't have antibody to rubella are also likely not to have antibody to mumps, so it is more cost-effective to give them a combination vaccine (there is no increased risk of side effects with MMR vaccine compared with rubella vaccine alone).

Vaccines for older children and adults. The same vaccine dosage is used for people of all ages.

Boosters (to enhance prior vaccinations). Boosters are not needed by anyone who has received 2 doses of MMR or MR vaccine.

How the Vaccine Is Given

Beneath the skin. Rubella vaccine is most often given as the combined MMR vaccine, as a single injection beneath the skin. The freeze-dried vaccine is mixed with distilled water prior to injection.

Although rubella vaccine is not as sensitive to sunlight and heat as measles vaccine, it should be refrigerated at 5–8°C (41–46°F) until it is used. If the vaccine virus dies before it is injected, it won't be able to stimulate the immune responses. Improper storage remains a problem and may be responsible for failures of the vaccine.

Schedule of Vaccination

Infants and children (under age 7). In Canada and the United States, the routine immunization schedule consists of 2 doses of rubella vaccine, given as the combined MMR vaccine. The first dose is given on or as soon after the first birthday as possible; the second dose is given at 4 to 6 years of age, before starting school. In a few Canadian provinces, the second dose is given at 18 months of age. Both schedules are effective.

Women. All women should have a blood test for immunity to rubella, preferably before their first pregnancy.
- *If the woman is not pregnant* and her blood lacks antibody to rubella, she should be immunized with rubella vaccine or MMR. Women should not become pregnant for 1 month after vaccination to allow immunity to develop.
- *If the woman is already pregnant* and the test reveals that she lacks antibody, vaccination should be delayed until immediately after delivery of the baby to avoid potential harm to the fetus [see below, *Reasons to avoid or delay rubella vaccine*].

Possible Side Effects of Rubella Vaccine

Mild. Infants rarely have any side effects after rubella vaccine. The frequency and severity of side effects after rubella vaccination increase with age, as does severity of the disease. Following vaccination, a few people develop mild fever, sore throat, headache, a rash and swollen glands, just like a mild case of rubella.

Most of these reactions are probably due to measles vaccine rather than rubella or mumps vaccines in the combined MMR vaccine; the frequency of reactions is the same in children receiving MMR or just measles vaccine.

Joint pain. The most significant side effect of the rubella vaccine is pain in the joints. This affects more adults than children. Following vaccination, about 1 in 4 adult women have some joint pain compared with less than 1 in 100 children (25% vs. 1%, respectively). The occurrence rate of joint pain is twice as high (in both children and women) with natural infection as with vaccination. The joints most often involved are those in the knees and fingers.

Arthritis (joint pain plus inflammation — redness, swelling and tenderness) is much less frequent. In about 10% of those with joint pain, the problem is severe enough to cause the person to miss a few days of work.

A recent study in Vancouver has raised doubt as to whether there really is an increased risk of arthritis in women after vaccination with rubella. Women who were susceptible to rubella were given either rubella vaccine or a placebo (in this case, an injection without vaccine). Actual arthritis was uncommon in both groups. However, the frequency of joint pain without signs of inflammation was the same in both groups following the injection.

Thrombocytopenia. Although it is rare, a few children develop a condition called thrombocytopenia (low platelets in the blood) after rubella vaccination. The decrease in platelets causes small hemorrhages and bruises in the skin. [For more information on this condition, see *Complications,* above.] However, the occurrence rate of thrombocytopenia is more than 10 times higher after natural infection than after rubella vaccination.

Reasons to Avoid or Delay Rubella Vaccine

Do not give. The National Advisory Committee on Immunization recognizes only one absolute reason not to give rubella vaccine: an allergic reaction (hives; swelling of face, lips or throat; wheezing; and/or shock [fall in blood pressure]) to neomycin (an antibiotic in the vaccine), to gelatin, or to a previous dose of rubella vaccine.

Do not delay. However, children with illnesses such as colds, ear infections or mild diarrhea should be vaccinated. The frequency of *minor infections* is so high after the first birthday that many children would never be vaccinated if such illnesses were considered valid reasons to delay vaccination! Children with colds, with or without fever, have the same immune responses and same rates of side effects as children without colds.

Rubella vaccine is recommended and has been shown to be safe for *children infected with HIV or AIDS who are not severely immunocompromised.*

Delay. Vaccination should be delayed for the reasons indicated below.

High fever. Vaccination should be delayed in anyone with a high fever to avoid confusing the fever or any other symptoms of illness with side effects of the vaccine.

Immunosuppression (lowered immune system). Although the current rubella vaccines have not been shown to cause harm in children who have suppression of the immune system due to underlying disease or medication, rubella vaccine should not be given to persons with severe disorders of the immune system. [See above for children infected with HIV or AIDS who are not severely immunocompromised.]

Recent injection with IG or other blood products. Immune globulin (IG) and other blood products may contain antibody to rubella virus that will interfere with the rubella vaccine. Vaccination must be delayed for 3 to 11 months, depending on the type and dose of IG or other blood product used.

Pregnancy. In Canada today, the risk of contracting rubella during pregnancy is so low that it is not worth the very low risk associated with having the vaccine. However, there have been no cases of congenital rubella syndrome in over 1,000 infants born to women who were vaccinated in the first 2 months of pregnancy. The babies were examined at birth and several times throughout the first year of life to be sure that they did not have congenital rubella syndrome.

There is no known risk of congenital rubella syndrome to the fetus as a result of rubella vaccination *after* the first 2 months of pregnancy. Therefore, rubella vaccination during pregnancy is no longer considered a reason for abortion.

But to avoid *any* risk to the fetus, it is recommended that pregnant women not be vaccinated with rubella or other live virus vaccines. It is safe, though, to vaccinate children of a woman who is pregnant; the virus contained in the rubella vaccine does not spread from person to person.

The Results of Vaccination

Long-lasting protection. The immune response to the RA27/3 rubella vaccine is very similar to the response after infection with the wild virus. The RA27/3 vaccine induces higher concentrations and also a broader range of antibodies than any of the other rubella vaccines. With both types of immunity (vaccine-induced and natural), antibody levels can fall below the "detectable" range. But most people with these unusually low antibody levels remain protected against infection because of immune memory cells.

For most people, vaccination results in long-lasting, if not lifelong, immunity.

Evidence that rubella vaccine works includes the following:
- Controlled studies have demonstrated that vaccination provides over 95% protection against rubella.
- There have been marked declines in the number of cases of rubella and congenital rubella syndrome in Canada and all other countries with infant immunization programs.

- The frequency of congenital rubella syndrome has decreased by over 99% in countries with the three-step vaccination program [see beginning of chapter, *After vaccine*]. Rare cases of rubella and congenital rubella syndrome have occurred even though the people had been vaccinated. No vaccine is 100% effective.

Summary

- Rubella is not a serious illness in children, however, it can cause death or severe malformation of the fetus if a pregnant woman acquires the infection during the first 20 weeks of her pregnancy.
- Rubella vaccine is very safe and causes no serious reactions in children.
- Routine immunization of children has markedly reduced the occurrence rate of rubella and congenital rubella syndrome.
- All children should be vaccinated against rubella in an effort to eradicate rubella virus and to put an end to congenital rubella syndrome.
- All women of child-bearing age should have a blood test to determine immunity to rubella, especially if they plan to become pregnant at any time. Those who are susceptible should receive the MMR vaccine.
- All pregnant women should be tested for immunity to rubella; those who are susceptible should be vaccinated as soon as possible after the birth of their child.

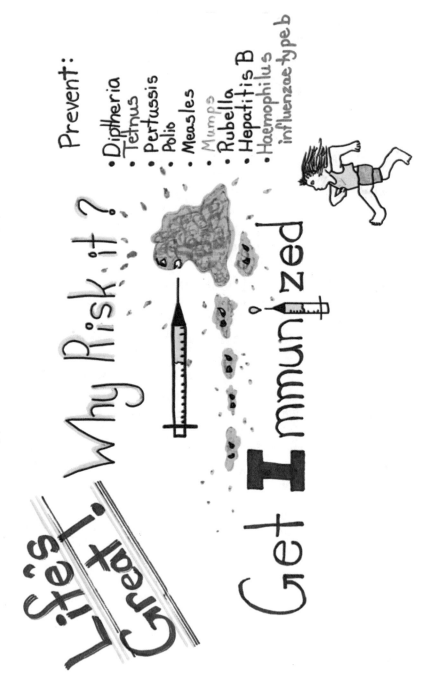

Life's Great!
Why Risk it?
Get Immunized

Prevent:
- Diptheria
- Tetnus
- Pertussis
- Polio
- Measles
- Mumps
- Rubella
- Hepatitis B
- Haemophilus influenzae type b

Laura Evans, Victoria, British Columbia

CHAPTER 11

Hepatitis B

Hepatitis B is an infection of the liver caused by a virus. The liver is the major chemical factory of the body:

- It completes the digestion of food begun in the stomach and intestines, changing the food into forms that can be used by various tissues.
- It stores sugar, fat and certain vitamins.
- It breaks down many chemicals and toxins so that they can be excreted by the body.

Half of the people who are infected with hepatitis B do not know they have the virus because they do not get sick (asymptomatic infection). Of this group, 10% are unable to get rid of the virus naturally (i.e., their immune system doesn't do its job). Because these people don't know they have the disease, they don't seek treatment and remain infected for life. They are called "chronic carriers." They may develop liver disease or liver cancer many years after becoming infected.

The other half of infected people become ill with fever, fatigue, loss of appetite, and yellow skin and eyes (jaundice). The illness may last weeks or months. Severe liver damage caused by infection may be fatal. Most people recover from the acute infection and are immune for life.

A History of Hepatitis B

Before Vaccine

The illness called hepatitis was described by Hippocrates more than 2,000 years ago. Studies during World War II showed that there were at least two different types of viral hepatitis. They were originally called infectious hepatitis and serum hepatitis, but are now called hepatitis A and B. [See Chapter 16 for a description of hepatitis A.]

Chronic carriers. Approximately 300 million people worldwide are chronic carriers of hepatitis B virus (i.e., the virus is in the person, but no symptoms appear for many years). Marked differences occur in the frequency of this type of infection among various parts of the world. In Canada, the United States and some other developed countries, about 1 person in 200 (0.5%) is a chronic carrier of the infection. In China, Southeast Asia and parts of Africa, about 1 person in 10 (10%) is a chronic carrier.

In Canada, it is estimated that 20,000 new hepatitis B infections (including both symptomatic and asymptomatic) occur every year. At least 10% of these result in chronic infection of the liver. Every year, chronic hepatitis B infection causes about 400 deaths from cirrhosis (scarring) of the liver and about 80 deaths from liver cancer. In China and other parts of the world where the rate of hepatitis B infection is quite high, cancer of the liver caused by hepatitis B is the most common type of cancer.

Blood tests detect infection. The development of sensitive and accurate blood tests to detect infection with hepatitis B virus in the 1970s enabled routine screening of blood donors. This resulted in a rapid and marked decrease in hepatitis B infections associated with transfusion of blood and blood products.

After Vaccine

The first hepatitis B vaccine became available in 1982. Subsequent changes in the method of making hepatitis B vaccine led to widespread availability and considerable reduction in cost. The vaccine has been shown to be very safe and very effective in preventing infection with hepatitis B virus.

In other countries. Mass immunization of all newborn infants in countries with high rates of chronic hepatitis B infection, such as Taiwan, has been extremely effective. Not only has the rate of infection of young children decreased by over 90%, but also the rate of liver cancer caused by hepatitis B infection and deaths from overwhelming hepatitis in infants have declined markedly.

In Canada. Routine immunization of pre-teen children in Canada has not yet been in operation long enough to produce a detectable decrease in the rate of hepatitis B infections.

The Germ

Researchers have identified the structure and chemical nature of the hepatitis B virus. The virus has an outer protein coat, called **hepatitis B surface antigen** (HBsAg for short), and an inner core protein that covers the DNA genes of the virus. Immunity to hepatitis B virus depends primarily on the antibody response to HBsAg.

How It Causes Illness

After the virus infects the liver cells, the fate of the virus depends on the immune response of the body. If the appropriate immune response develops, immune white blood cells attack the infected liver cells and destroy them. In the process, the virus is also destroyed.

Chronic infection. About 5–10% of adults infected with hepatitis B do not have the normal immune response to the virus and are unable to get rid of the infected cells. The virus persists and continues to multiply in the liver cells. Ultimately, the chronic infection causes damage to the liver, which may lead to scarring of the liver (known as cirrhosis) and death from liver failure.

Chronic infection may also result in cancer of the liver, which is almost always fatal, too. Many years may pass between the infection and onset of illness due to chronic liver disease. During this time, the person may not be aware of the infection because no symptoms develop.

Those at greatest risk. The risk of developing chronic infection with hepatitis B is much higher in persons with an undeveloped immune system (such as in infants and young children) and in persons with underlying medical problems affecting the immune system. More than 90% of infants who acquire hepatitis B at birth from their infected mothers will develop chronic infection.

How Hepatitis B Is Spread

Contaminated body fluids. Chronic carriers remain contagious for as long as the virus persists in the liver, usually for life. For chronic carriers and those acutely ill with hepatitis B, the virus is present in the blood and certain other body fluids, including semen, secretions in the genital tract, and breast milk. Other body fluids that become contaminated with blood may also have hepatitis B virus in them.

Not ordinary daily contact. Hepatitis B virus is not spread in the general population by ordinary daily contact. It cannot be breathed in, as can most of the other infections described in this book. The Table below lists the most common means of transmission of this virus.

TABLE 11.1

The most common ways that hepatitis B virus spreads

MEANS OF INFECTION	EXAMPLES
Penetration of the skin with virus-contaminated equipment or fluids	• Transfusion of infected blood or infected blood product • Injection with contaminated needles and syringes • Tattooing and body piercing with contaminated equipment • Hemodialysis (filtering of the blood) with contaminated equipment or fluids
Exposure of membranes of mouth or genital tract to blood or to body fluids containing blood	• Sexual activity or intimate physical contact with infected person • Newborn exposed to blood of infected mother before or during birth • Breastfeeding by infected mother • Sharing of personal hygiene items (e.g., toothbrushes, razors) with infected person

In Canada, the two most common means of spread are sexual activity and shared needles (by drug users). The infection rate is highest among older teenagers and young adults. Infection of infants born to infected mothers still occurs, but the rate is decreasing for two reasons:
- women are now being tested for hepatitis B infection during pregnancy;
- the newborn babies of women who are infected can be protected as soon as possible after birth with vaccine plus hepatitis B immune globulin [see below, *Treatment*].

The Illness

The incubation period of hepatitis B (time between infection and the onset of symptoms) varies between 6 weeks and 6 months. This is much longer than the incubation period of most other infections.

Symptoms of acute illness. Half of infected patients develop an acute illness. Those who do become sick following infection with hepatitis B may have symptoms for up to a week before jaundice appears [see description of this condition, below]. Symptoms may include fever, headache, aches and pains, loss of appetite, nausea and vomiting. Most patients also have weakness and fatigue.

In some patients, *jaundice* is the first sign of illness. The urine becomes dark. Over the next few days, the skin and white of the eyes turn yellow. The bowel movements usually become light or grey in colour. This condition occurs because the liver can no longer excrete bile normally.

Recovery. The illness is usually milder in children than in adults. The duration of illness varies widely, from a few days to many weeks. The symptoms and jaundice clear gradually. Most older children, adolescents and adults infected with hepatitis B virus make a complete recovery, develop lifelong immunity and do not get chronic liver disease.

Asymptomatic infection. Of all persons infected with hepatitis B, half develop no symptoms at all, even though blood tests confirm infection. Most of those who don't know they are infected develop the appropriate immune response and are able to rid their body of the infection. But some people (10% of those infected) are unable to get rid of the virus. They are called *chronic carriers*. The persistence of the virus in the liver leads to *chronic liver disease*. [See *Complications*, below.]

Complications

Of acute infection. In about 1 out of 100 acute infections, the illness is so severe that the liver stops working and there is a high risk of *death*.

Of chronic infection. The most common complication is persistent infection of the liver, or *chronic hepatitis*. The chronic infection is usually without any noticeable symptoms for years. The only indication of a chronic condition in the early stages can be found in blood tests. They can reveal abnormal function of the liver and persistence of hepatitis B virus.

Eventually, loss of appetite, weight loss, abdominal pain, fluid retention and bleeding problems may develop as the result of liver damage.

Chronic infection over time often leads to widespread scarring of the liver. Severe scarring may result in *liver failure and death*. Chronic infection with hepatitis B virus can also cause *cancer of the liver*. The risk of developing chronic infection depends on the age of the person at the time of infection [see Table below].

TABLE 11.2

The risk of developing chronic hepatitis B infection, by age

AGE AT TIME OF INFECTION	RISK OF DEVELOPING CHRONIC INFECTION (%)
Newborn	90
1 to 5 years	20–30
Over 5 years	5–10

Diagnosis

Symptoms of jaundice, loss of appetite, nausea, vomiting, abdominal pain, and blood tests showing abnormal liver function suggest viral infection of the liver. Infection with hepatitis B virus is confirmed by blood tests.

Treatment

Acute infection. No treatment is available for the acute infection.

Chronic infection. A drug called **interferon**, which is given by injection, has been used to treat chronic hepatitis B infection, but it is not always successful.

Prevention of infection. A special preparation of immune globulin, called **hepatitis B immune globulin (HBIG)**, is available for prevention of infection following exposure of a non-immune person to hepatitis B virus. HBIG is given by injection into muscle. It contains a large amount of antibody against hepatitis B virus. The antibodies coat the virus particles, enabling white blood cells to destroy the virus before it can damage the liver.

How is HBIG made? It is made from plasma of blood donors who have high concentrations of antibody against hepatitis B, because of either vaccination or previous infection with the virus. Blood tests confirm that the donors have completely recovered from the infection and do not have any evidence of chronic infection. The donors are also tested to be sure that they are not infected with hepatitis C virus or HIV (the AIDS virus).

Is HBIG safe? Current methods of testing blood from volunteer donors and of preparing HBIG ensure that there is no risk of acquiring HIV, hepatitis B or hepatitis C from this product. Other than pain at the injection site, there are no significant reactions to HBIG.

Does HBIG work? For maximum effect, HBIG should be administered as soon as possible after exposure, preferably within 48 hours. HBIG is approximately 75% effective in preventing infection. Persons exposed to hepatitis B virus should receive hepatitis B vaccine as well as HBIG.

Who should have HBIG?

Although HBIG is not 100% effective in preventing infection, it is recommended for those who have not been fully immunized *and* who have been exposed to hepatitis B virus under the following circumstances:

* accidental needle-stick or other injury;
* sexual activity with an infected person;
* an infant born to an infected mother.

Post-infection. Persons who recover from an infection with hepatitis B virus develop lifelong immunity.

The Vaccine

Type of Vaccine

Purified viral protein. Hepatitis B vaccine is unique compared with other vaccines in that the vaccine has been developed even though the virus cannot yet be grown in the laboratory. Hepatitis B vaccine consists of the protein that forms the outer coat of the virus particle. The protein is highly purified and contains no other part of the virus. The vaccine cannot cause hepatitis B infection because there are no whole virus particles in the vaccine.

How Hepatitis B Vaccine Is Made

Process. The vaccines currently used in Canada are prepared by recombinant (meaning "formed by recombination") gene technology. The gene of the hepatitis B virus that makes the hepatitis B surface protein has been isolated and transferred into yeast cells. The yeast cells function like small factories. When they multiply, they make large quantities of hepatitis B surface protein. The protein is extracted from the culture fluid that the yeast is grown in, and then purified. The vaccine contains less than 50 mg (0.05 g) of yeast protein per dose.

Additives. The purified vaccine is mixed with aluminum hydroxide to enhance the immune response. Current vaccines *do not* contain thimerosal, a mercury-containing preservative. The hepatitis B vaccine produced *before 2001* contained 0.005% thimerosal (50 parts per million).

Testing. Tests for potency (effectiveness), toxicity and sterility are carried out on all batches of vaccine, by both the manufacturer and the Bureau of Biologics and Radiopharmaceuticals [see Chapter 2].

Available Forms of Hepatitis B Vaccine

Combinations. Hepatitis B vaccine is available alone or in combination with hepatitis A vaccine. The combined product is particularly useful for travellers going to parts of the world where both infections are common.

Vaccines for older children and adults. The quantity of the doses given varies with age of the recipient and with vaccines from different manufacturers.

Boosters (to enhance prior vaccinations). Boosters are not recommended after completion of a series of injections, except for persons with underlying diseases that interfere with normal immune responses (e.g., chronic kidney disease requiring dialysis).

How the Vaccine Is Given

Into muscle. Hepatitis B vaccine is administered by injection into the muscle of the leg or arm. It is important that this vaccine is injected into the muscle rather than into the overlying tissue beneath the skin (subcutaneous tissue). Injection into muscle causes much milder local reaction (e.g., redness, swelling) than injection under the skin.

Schedule of Vaccination

At this time, **there is no universal schedule for routine immunization** with hepatitis B vaccine. [See Text Box below for persons who should receive the vaccine for prevention of hepatitis B infection.]

The *most common schedule* consists of 3 doses of vaccine given over a 6-month period. The first dose is given; 1 month later, the second dose is given; 5 months later, the third dose is given. A two-dose schedule for adolescents is also possible.

Who should be vaccinated?

- Newborns of infected mothers
- All children prior to adolescence
- Persons at increased risk of infection [see below, *The results of vaccination,* for details]

The **duration of protection** is not yet known. It does, however, last at least 10 years, and probably much longer.

Possible Side Effects of Hepatitis B Vaccine

Mild. Millions of doses of hepatitis B vaccine have been given over the past 20 years. Pain and tenderness at the site of the injection occur after about 15% of vaccinations. The soreness is mild and lasts less than 24 hours. Carefully controlled studies have found that other symptoms, such as fever, headache, muscle aches and pain, nausea, vomiting, loss of appetite and fatigue, occur at the same rates in persons who receive the vaccine as in those who are given a placebo (in this case, an injection containing no vaccine).

Allergic reactions are rare, occurring after less than 1% of vaccinations. Such reactions may be caused by allergy to yeast proteins in the vaccine.

Safe vaccine. The various hepatitis B vaccines have been shown to be very safe. There is no risk of infection with hepatitis B or any other virus from the vaccine.

Unfounded claims. There is no valid scientific evidence that hepatitis B vaccine causes multiple sclerosis (MS). Patients with MS are not at risk of exacerbation of their symptoms when vaccinated with hepatitis B vaccine.

Reasons to Avoid or Delay Hepatitis B Vaccine

Do not give. The National Advisory Committee on Immunization recognizes only one reason not to give hepatitis B vaccination: an anaphylactic reaction to a previous dose of the vaccine. Anaphylaxis is a severe allergic reaction involving one or more of the following: swelling of face or lips, difficulty breathing or shock (fall in blood pressure).

Do not delay. The vaccine can be given during pregnancy if necessary.

The Results of Vaccination

In general. Overall, hepatitis B vaccine is very effective. Over 95% of those vaccinated develop antibody and are protected against infection with hepatitis B virus. Those who do become infected despite vaccination appear to be protected against developing chronic hepatitis B infection. The duration of protection is not yet known. It does, however, last at least 10 years, and probably much longer. For now, booster doses of vaccine are not necessary in most cases.

First strategy. When the vaccine first became available in 1982, it was recommended for persons at increased risk of infection with hepatitis B, including:
- health-care workers and others at risk of infection because of frequent exposure to blood as part of their occupation (e.g., doctors, nurses, dentists);
- persons with underlying diseases that require treatment with blood or blood products (e.g., hemophilia and chronic kidney failure treated with dialysis);
- infants whose mothers have chronic hepatitis B infection;
- persons living with someone with chronic hepatitis B infection;
- those travelling to areas with high rates of hepatitis B infection.

This approach of targeting high-risk groups has been very effective in reducing the number of infections in persons in the first three groups listed above. However, there was little or no effect on the overall rate of hepatitis B infections in Canada or the United States in the decade following the introduction of the vaccine. Part of the reason for this was that many people in the high-risk groups had not been vaccinated.

Current strategy. To control hepatitis B infection, medical authorities in both Canada and the United States now recommend immunization of all children with the vaccine. Italy, New Zealand and several Asian countries have already introduced routine vaccination of all infants.

The benefit of routine vaccination of all infants has now been clearly demonstrated in Taiwan. Not only has the frequency of infection in newborns and children decreased markedly, but there has also been a significant decrease in liver cancer due to hepatitis B infection.

The current strategy for prevention of hepatitis B infection in Canada, which focuses on three groups, is as follows:

1. Test all pregnant women for chronic infection with hepatitis B so that *newborns of infected mothers* can be protected as soon as possible after birth with vaccine plus hepatitis B immune globulin (HBIG) [see above, *Treatment*].

2. Vaccinate *all children prior to adolescence* so that they are protected before becoming sexually active. School vaccination programs have begun in all provinces and territories in Canada. Some provinces also vaccinate all infants.

3. Vaccinate *those at increased risk of infection* because of
   a. occupation (e.g., doctors, nurses and dentists; medical, dental and nursing students; other health care workers);
   b. underlying medical problems requiring frequent transfusion of blood or blood products;
   c. behaviours such as injectable drug use;
   d. close daily proximity to and/or contact with someone who has chronic hepatitis B infection (e.g., living in a household with an infected person).

Vaccinating children. The decision to recommend vaccination of all children was based on these facts: the vaccine is safe and effective, and the vaccination program is affordable. It costs more to treat chronic liver disease caused by hepatitis B than to vaccinate all children.

Infants. New Brunswick and British Columbia have elected to vaccinate all infants as well as school-age children. Routine infant vaccination programs will be more widely accepted if a suitable combination vaccine can be developed (i.e., one that does not result in increased reactions or decreased antibody responses). The ideal combination would include vaccines against diphtheria, tetanus, pertussis, polio, Hib and hepatitis B.

School-age children. Most provinces and territories in Canada recommend routine vaccination of school-age children rather than infants for the following reasons:
- The rate of hepatitis B infection is very low in children under 12 years of age, but begins to rise rapidly after 15 years of age.
- A combination product (diphtheria, tetanus, pertussis, polio, Hib and hepatitis B vaccines) is not yet available.

Evidence that hepatitis B vaccine works includes the following:
- Controlled trials demonstrated that hepatitis B vaccine is over 90% effective in preventing infection by means of sexual transmission.
- Controlled trials demonstrated that hepatitis B vaccine administered to newborns whose mothers have chronic hepatitis infection is over 95% effective in preventing infection of the newborn.
- Routine immunization of all newborns in Taiwan resulted in a marked drop in the rates of hepatitis B-related infant infections and liver cancer.

Summary

- Hepatitis B disease is a major health problem worldwide: more than 3 million people have chronic infection.
- Chronic liver disease and liver cancer resulting from hepatitis B infection cause many deaths worldwide.
- Hepatitis B vaccine is highly purified and has been shown to be safe and effective.

- Routine vaccination of children offers the opportunity to eradicate hepatitis B and prevent a common type of cancer.
- School vaccination programs in Canada have been very successful in that they have reached well over 90% of eligible children.
- Infant vaccination programs may become routine once a combination vaccine is developed.

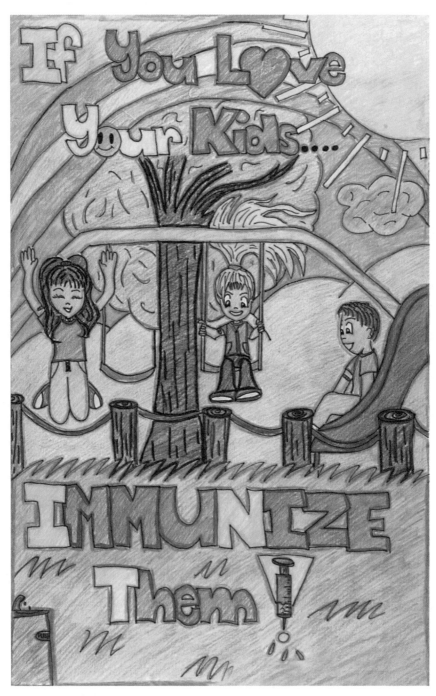

Shaunna B. Salangsang, Winnipeg, Manitoba

CHAPTER 12

Influenza

Influenza is a virus that causes epidemics of flu, bronchitis (infection of the airways) and pneumonia (infection of the lungs) every year in the late fall or winter. Although the illnesses caused by influenza virus may be identical to illnesses caused by cold viruses, the influenza virus is much more dangerous. It can cause severe illness and death.

Influenza can also cause very large epidemics. No other virus causing acute respiratory illness can spread so rapidly to large numbers of the population. Up to 20% of people can be infected with influenza virus during a single epidemic. Laboratory tests can determine whether influenza is the cause of illness.

Whenever outbreaks of influenza occur, there is an increase in the hospitalization and death rates of infants (children less than 12 months old) and elderly persons (age 65 and over). Most deaths involve elderly persons and those who have serious heart or lung disease.

The influenza vaccine is commonly called "the flu shot."

A History of Influenza

Before Vaccine

Influenza virus was first isolated in humans in 1933. Because of its unique ability to infect many people over a short period of time, influenza has been identified in historical records as having caused 299 epidemics between 1173 and 1875.

A worldwide epidemic (called a pandemic) was first described in 1580. As the rate and extent of international travel increased, so too did the spread of influenza. Major pandemics have occurred in:
- 1889–90 ("Russian Flu" with an estimated 250,000 deaths in Europe, and a death total worldwide of two or three times that number);
- 1918 (20 million deaths worldwide, 450,000 deaths in the United States alone);
- 1957 ("Asian Flu" with 60,000 deaths); and
- 1968 ("Hong Kong Flu" with 50 million cases and 33,000 deaths).

Each year since 1980, there have been 130,000 to 170,000 hospitalizations and 10,000 to 40,000 deaths caused by influenza. Every year, it infects 10–20% of the population in the United States. Over 90% of deaths occur among the elderly.

After Vaccine

Until recently, influenza vaccination programs in Canada and the United States have been directed primarily at high-risk groups: that is, those who are at increased risk of severe illness or death because of age or underlying medical condition [see Text Box later in this Chapter]. Because of continual changes in the influenza A viruses (the strains that cause most infections and all large epidemics of influenza), the vaccine must be given every year. (Influenza B viruses also change, but much more slowly than influenza A.)

For this reason, in all parts of Canada except Ontario [see *The results of vaccination*, later in this Chapter], influenza vaccination has not been used on a routine basis for all persons. Rather, the goal of influenza vaccination programs has been to reduce deaths and severe illness from influenza among those at highest risk of the disease, namely, the elderly and those (of any age) with chronic medical conditions. These vaccination programs have reduced hospitalization rates by 50–70% and deaths due to influenza by an average of 85% in the elderly. At the time of writing, individuals must pay for the vaccine themselves in most provinces and territories.

The Germ

Influenza A strains more common. There are two major groups of influenza virus: A and B. Influenza A strains cause most infections and all large epidemics of influenza. Influenza A strains are divided into subtypes on the basis of two proteins on the surface of the virus, called hemagglutinin (H) and neuraminidase (N).

Immunity against influenza. Immunity to these two surface proteins, especially to H, protects against infection and reduces the severity of illness if infection does occur. Immunity to influenza is very specific. Infection with one subtype of influenza A induces immunity only to that subtype and provides little or no protection against other subtypes and none against influenza B.

An ever-changing virus. Almost every year, minor changes occur in the proteins that coat *the influenza A virus*. The changes are the result of mutations in the genes for H and/or N. These slight changes pose a problem for the immune system: because the proteins coating the virus are different each year, the immune system will not recognize the virus and will treat it as a "new" one (i.e., immune memory established in previous years will not activate immune responses for this altered virus). This is the reason why infection with influenza occurs in people again and again, year after year. [For more information on immune memory, see Chapter 1.]

Similar changes in *influenza B strains* occur much more slowly. The ability of the virus to keep changing the proteins on its surface is the key to its success in causing epidemics. Immune memory allows our body to recognize when it is infected with influenza. However, the memory cells trigger the production of antibodies to strains with which the body has been infected in the past. This process has been termed "original antigenic sin."

These antibodies are often not effective against the new strains of influenza because of the altered surface proteins. Essentially, no one can establish immune memory to the virus, so it spreads through populations like wildfire.

Changes lead to global epidemics. Influenza virus has another mechanism to escape attack by the human immune system, in addition to mutations of H and N genes. By means of what is called *"antigenic shift,"* influenza A viruses can acquire an entirely new and different H or N gene, usually from an animal strain of influenza A.

Because the new H or N protein differs completely from that on the surface of existing strains causing infections in the population, very few people will have any immunity to the new strain. Such changes may lead to pandemics of influenza.

How It Causes Illness

The respiratory tract is the major target of influenza virus. After infected droplets are inhaled or reach the nose via contaminated fingers, the virus infects and multiplies in the surface cells lining the nose and pharynx (the space connecting the mouth to the esophagus, which is the tube that connects to the stomach).

By unknown mechanisms, the virus ultimately kills these cells. The lining of the nose, throat, trachea (the airway connecting the larynx or voice box to the bronchi), bronchi (large air passages of the lungs) and bronchioles (small divisions of the larger bronchi) are damaged to varying degrees.

How Influenza Is Spread

Direct contact, airborne, contaminated objects. The illness induced by influenza virus ensures that it spreads widely. Large amounts of infectious virus contaminate respiratory secretions. The infected person releases these secretions into the air by coughing, sneezing, talking and singing. The virus is relatively stable within small airborne particles, so it can spread to others through the air.

It also spreads directly from person to person when contaminated droplets are released or by touching surfaces contaminated with the virus and then touching the virus-laden fingers to one's nose or eyes.

Highly contagious. Influenza is very contagious. The disease spreads rapidly because the incubation period (time from exposure to the virus to the start of infection) is short (only 1 to 2 days) and because illness is often relatively mild in school-age children, allowing them to continue to go to school even though they are highly contagious. School-age children are most responsible for the spread of influenza throughout the community.

Duration of contagiousness. Contagiousness persists for 3 to 5 days after the onset of illness.

The Illness

Influenza infection results in a wide range of illness:
- infection without any symptoms;
- common cold-like illness with or without fever;
- typical "flu" with sudden onset of fever, headache, aches and pains, fatigue, sore throat and cough;
- high fever (greater than 40°C/104°F) without other symptoms, especially in infants and young children;
- croup (fever, harsh barking cough, breathing difficulty) in children less than 2 years of age;
- fever and convulsions in infants and young children;

- fever, vomiting, abdominal pain and diarrhea, with or without respiratory symptoms, especially in infants and young children.

Symptoms. The damage to the respiratory tract caused by influenza results in runny nose, sore throat and cough. The generalized symptoms of fever, headache, aches and pains, fatigue and physical exhaustion are not the result of spread of the virus through the body, but rather the result of the intense response of body defences to the infection.

Influenza is unique in the rapidity of onset of symptoms. Individuals feel well and then are suddenly (over a few hours) overcome by headache, aches and pains, and intense fatigue.

Complications

Pneumonia (infection of the lungs) is the most common complication of influenza, caused either by the virus itself or by bacteria invading areas damaged by the virus. Pneumonia is the most common cause of death from influenza, especially in those with chronic heart and lung conditions.

Other complications include:
- *febrile seizures* (those caused by fever) in infants and young children;
- *myositis* (severe muscle inflammation) in children with influenza B infection, primarily affecting the calf muscles of both legs;
- *myocarditis* (inflammation of the heart muscle), which may lead to abnormal heart rhythm, heart failure and death;
- *encephalitis* (inflammation of the brain), which may lead to brain damage and death;
- *Reye's syndrome*, a condition that causes damage to the brain and liver. This disorder has become quite rare because acetylsalicylic acid (ASA, aspirin) is no longer recommended for use in children to control fever.

Diagnosis

Diagnosis of influenza requires laboratory tests because the illness is similar to that caused by many other respiratory viruses. Different tests examine different aspects of the virus:

- Growing a culture of the virus (obtained by throat swab) can identify the virus; it takes 3 to 4 days to process.
- Blood tests can detect a rise in influenza antibody in the blood 21 days after onset of illness.
- New rapid methods detect influenza A proteins or influenza genes in respiratory secretions within a few hours.

There are two main benefits of rapid confirmation of influenza A infection:

- It enables prompt use of drugs that are active against influenza, but not other viruses.
- It allows more rapid implementation of measures to reduce the spread of the virus to others, especially within hospitals, nursing homes, retirement homes, and other institutions that care for elderly persons.

Treatment

New medication. Two types of medication are now available to treat influenza infections. They are oral drugs that interfere with multiplication of the virus in the body. To have any effect, they must be started within 48 hours of onset of symptoms. The medicines

- shorten the duration of fever and respiratory symptoms by about 50%;
- reduce the amount of virus in respiratory secretions;
- shorten the duration of contagiousness so that spread of the virus is also reduced.

Prevention. The medications can also be used to prevent infection with influenza, but must be given before exposure to the virus occurs. Medication is usually given for the duration of the influenza season. Preventive use of the medications is recommended primarily for persons at high risk of serious illness or death from influenza who either have not yet been vaccinated or are not expected to have a protective immune response to the vaccine because of underlying medical conditions [see Text Box below for a list of these conditions].

The Vaccine

Type of Vaccine

Influenza vaccine is a **killed virus vaccine**. To make the vaccine, different virus strains are used each year to match (as closely as possible) the strains causing outbreaks of disease around the world. The virus is grown in fertilized chicken eggs and then purified. The purified virus is then treated with a detergent. This treatment breaks the virus into smaller pieces, which are further purified. The resulting product is called a *split virus vaccine*.

The vaccine does not cause the recipient to get the flu. Because there is no live virus in the vaccine, vaccination cannot lead to spread of influenza.

Due to the continual changes in the H and N proteins of influenza A virus, the strains used to make the vaccine have to be updated annually. The World Health Organization has established a network of laboratories around the world for the purpose of isolating and identifying the changes in influenza viruses.

The decision about which strains to include in the vaccine is made in February of each year. Manufacturers then have sufficient time to produce the vaccine for the influenza season, the following autumn.

How Influenza Vaccine Is Made

Process. Influenza viruses are grown in fertilized chicken eggs. Since each egg yields only 1 or 2 doses of vaccine, tens of millions of eggs are used each year to produce the vaccine for Canada and the United States. The vaccine production process varies between manufacturers, but involves concentration and purification by physical processes such as centrifugation or chromatography, and chemical inactivation.

The inactivated virus particles are further treated to produce the split virus vaccine. To do this, the intact virus particles are treated with detergents to split the virus and purified by physical processes to remove almost all of the internal virus proteins. Split product vaccines contain residual egg proteins [see *Reasons to avoid or delay influenza vaccine,* below].

Additives. Although antibiotics are used in the production process, none are detectable in the final vaccine. Depending on the manufacturer, the vaccine may contain small amounts of formaldehyde (less than 0.1 mg/dose), gelatin (0.25 mg/dose) and thimerosal (0.05 mg/dose). Thimerosal is a mercury-containing preservative used to prevent bacterial contamination of the vaccine. There is no evidence that the very small amount of mercury present in the vaccine causes any harm. [See Chapter 17, Questions 16 and 19, for more information on thimerosal.]

Testing. Tests for potency (effectiveness), toxicity and sterility are carried out on all batches of vaccine, by both the manufacturer and the Bureau of Biologics and Radiopharmaceuticals [see Chapter 2].

Available Forms of Influenza Vaccine

Combinations. Influenza vaccine is available only on its own; it is not combined with any other vaccines.

Vaccines for older children and adults. There is no difference in the dosage of vaccines for infants (children less than 12 months of age), older children and adults.

Boosters (to enhance prior vaccinations). Boosters are required every year in order to maintain immunity for two reasons: the relatively short duration of immunity induced by the vaccine and the continual changes in the influenza viruses.

How the Vaccine Is Given

Influenza vaccine is given by injection into muscle.

Who Should Receive Influenza Vaccine?

Target groups. The primary goal of the influenza immunization programs in Canada and the United States is to reduce illness and death rates from influenza. To achieve this goal, the programs have concentrated on vaccinating three groups:

- those who are at high risk of serious illness or death from influenza (see Text Box below);
- those who are capable of spreading influenza to people at high risk, such as health-care workers and household contacts of high-risk persons;
- those who provide essential community services during influenza epidemics (e.g., doctors, nurses, ambulance drivers, police, firefighters).

Persons at increased risk of severe or fatal illness from influenza

- Adults and children with chronic heart or lung disorders that require regular medical care
- Residents (of any age) of nursing homes and other chronic care facilities
- People 65 years of age or older
- Adults and children* with chronic medical conditions:
  - diabetes
  - cancer
  - disorders of the immune system
  - kidney disorders
  - anemia
  - HIV infection and AIDS
- Children (6 months to 18 years of age) who must take acetylsalicylic acid (ASA or aspirin) on a daily basis

* Whether children with chronic medical conditions are at increased risk of severe influenza is controversial.

General population. Recent studies have demonstrated that the hospitalization rates due to influenza are as high for infants as for the elderly. Moreover, illness among healthy children and adults under age 65 is so widespread that the costs associated with influenza infection are tremendous.

Therefore the National Advisory Committee on Immunization [see Chapter 2, under *Making recommendations on vaccine use*] for 2001–02 recommends the following: healthy adults and their children who wish to protect themselves from influenza should be encouraged to receive the vaccine. [See *Reasons to avoid or delay influenza vaccine*, below, for exceptions within the general population.]

Schedule of Vaccination

Infants less than 6 months old. Immunization is not recommended for infants less than 6 months of age because the influenza vaccines currently available do not induce adequate antibody responses in young infants.

Children between 6 months and 9 years of age who have never received a dose of influenza vaccine require 2 doses of split virus vaccine, given at least 4 weeks apart. A second dose is not needed if the child has received 1 or more doses of vaccine in a previous influenza season.

For those aged 9 and over, only 1 dose of split virus vaccine is required, regardless of their influenza history.

Duration of protection. Protection against the virus lasts about 1 year. Those at risk should receive the vaccine every year to stay protected.

Possible Side Effects of Influenza Vaccine

Local and mild reactions. With the split virus vaccines, side effects occur at similar rates in children and adults. About two-thirds of vaccine recipients have soreness at the injection site for 1 to 2 days. Mild fever, muscle aches and pains, and fatigue, lasting 1 to 2 days, occur less frequently than local reactions.

Allergic reactions (hives; swelling of face, lips or throat; wheezing; and/or shock [fall in blood pressure]) after influenza vaccine are extremely rare.

In MS patients. Influenza vaccine has not been shown to cause exacerbation (worsening) of symptoms in patients with multiple sclerosis (MS).

Guillain-Barré syndrome, a neurologic disorder with muscle paralysis, has been reported after influenza vaccination, especially after use of the Swine Flu vaccine in 1978. In recent years, the risk of Guillain-Barré syndrome has been estimated to be 1.1 additional cases above the background rate (i.e., the rate in unvaccinated persons) for every 1 million influenza vaccinations. The risks of influenza are *much* greater.

New adverse event, ORS. During 2000–01, there were 960 reports in Canada of a new adverse event occurring after influenza vaccine, called oculo-respiratory syndrome (ORS). The symptoms of ORS developed within 2 to 24 hours after vaccination and included:
• red eyes;
• respiratory symptoms (e.g., cough, sore throat, difficulty breathing, wheezing or chest tightness);
• swelling of the face.

The symptoms were mild and cleared within 48 hours in most cases. Three-quarters of cases occurred in adult women, 30 to 59 years of age. Less than 10% occurred in children. ORS has occurred at similar rates after both vaccines available in Canada. (The vaccines are the same, just made by different manufacturers.) The cause of ORS is not yet known.

Testing. Before the vaccines were licensed for use in 2001–02, tests were done to make sure that no influenza vaccines caused ORS.

Reasons to Avoid or Delay Influenza Vaccine

Do not give. Influenza vaccine is not recommended for *infants less than 6 months of age* because of ineffectiveness in this age group, or for *persons who have an allergy to thimerosal* (a preservative used in contact lens solutions and the flu vaccine).

Pregnant and breastfeeding women. Influenza vaccine is safe for pregnant women at all stages of pregnancy and for breastfeeding mothers. Some studies have shown that there is an increased risk of complications from influenza during pregnancy. However, the National Advisory Committee on Immunization has concluded that there is insufficient evidence at present to recommend routine influenza vaccination of otherwise healthy women who are pregnant or breastfeeding during influenza season.

Persons allergic to eggs. Influenza vaccine is grown in chicken eggs and contains trace amounts of egg protein. Therefore, the vaccine should not be given to persons known to have severe allergic reactions or anaphylaxis after eating eggs, including hives, swelling of the mouth and throat, difficulty in breathing, and/or low blood pressure.

Do not delay. Vaccination should not be deferred or delayed because of minor illnesses, such as the common cold, with or without fever. Such infections do not increase the risk of side effects and do not interfere with the immune response to vaccination.

Delay. Moderate to severe illness, with or without fever, is a reason to delay influenza immunization. This precaution should be taken to avoid adding any side effects of the vaccine on top of the effects of the illness itself.

The Results of Vaccination

If the strains of virus in the vaccine match the wild strain, the vaccine will prevent infection in about 70% of healthy children and adults. For those who become infected despite vaccination, illness is milder than in those who haven't been vaccinated.

In older persons. Vaccination is especially important for older persons because they are at greatest risk of severe illness and death from influenza. Even though vaccination is less effective in persons over

65 years than in younger adults, it does reduce the severity of the illness in this age group. Hospitalization due to influenza is 50–70% lower and influenza-related deaths are about 85% lower in vaccinated than in unvaccinated elderly persons.

Year-to-year changes, short protection. Protection against the virus lasts only about 1 year. Because of the brief duration of protection as well as the frequent changes in influenza viruses, the vaccine must be given every year to those at risk to maintain protection. The need for annual vaccination makes this vaccine somewhat burdensome for routine use in healthy children and young adults.

Trial program. Ontario introduced a universal influenza immunization program in 2000 under which the vaccine is available free of charge to all Ontario residents. It is too early to assess the impact of this program.

Evidence that influenza vaccine works includes:
- reduced influenza infection and illness rates in vaccinated children and adults;
- reduced hospitalization and death rates in vaccinated persons aged 65 and over;
- decreased influenza rates in vaccinated health-care workers during influenza epidemics.

Outbreaks in other countries. In Japan, immunization of school-age children was compulsory for a number of years. After the compulsory program was discontinued, immunization rates dropped to very low levels. Since then, there has been a striking increase in the rates of influenza and deaths from influenza in Japan, especially among infants (children less than 12 months old) and the elderly (people aged 65 and over).

The rise in influenza rates after stopping the compulsory program strongly suggests that routine immunization of schoolchildren reduced the spread of influenza viruses in Japan.

Summary

- Influenza is a rapid-spreading virus that can lead to severe illness and death.
- Influenza vaccine is very safe and effective. Unfortunately, it is least effective in people aged 65 and over — one of the groups most at risk from influenza. However, the effects of influenza are considerably lessened in people who become infected despite being vaccinated.
- New influenza vaccines must be developed each year to match the ever-changing composition of the virus. Vaccines that provided immunity one year are ineffective the next.
- Routine vaccination of those at increased risk of severe disease or death from influenza is the most effective way of reducing the impact of influenza epidemics.
- Most Canadian provinces and territories have programs to provide influenza vaccination to the elderly (especially residents of nursing homes) and to those living in other chronic care facilities.
- There is a need to broaden the scope of the programs in all provinces and territories to include any children and adults under 65 years of age who are at increased risk of severe illness from influenza.

Why be sick and Grumpy

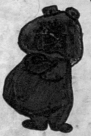

When you can be Healthy and Happy

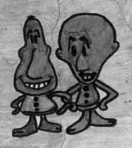

Get your immunizations today.

Laurens Philipsen, Patricia, Alberta

CHAPTER 13

Pneumococcal Disease

The bacterium called pneumococcus (or *Streptococcus pneumoniae*) is the most common cause of bacterial infections in children and a frequent cause of infections in adults. There are more than 90 strains (or serotypes) of pneumococci. Because the strains are all different, the immune system must develop a specific immune response to each one. Certain strains are much more common causes of disease than others: over 90% of all pneumococcal infections are caused by just 23 serotypes.

Until recently, all strains of pneumococci responded to penicillin and other antibiotics. However, an ever-increasing proportion of strains have become resistant to penicillin and other common antibiotics, making treatment more difficult. For example, even with modern treatment and intensive care, about 20% of patients with meningitis caused by pneumococcal bacteria die; a similar proportion of survivors suffer brain damage and deafness.

Infections involving these bacteria occur most frequently in the first 2 years of life, but they can occur at any age.

A History of Pneumococcal Disease

Before Vaccine

The first vaccine against the pneumococcal bacteria was developed in the late 1940s but was never widely used. (The introduction of penicillin right after World War II made the vaccine appear to be obsolete.) It consisted of polysaccharides (or complex sugars) from only 4 of the serotypes (strains) that cause pneumococcal infections.

Until the introduction of the conjugate vaccine in 2001 [see *After vaccine*, below], about 500,000 cases of pneumococcal disease occurred every year in Canada. Of these, approximately 65 children less than 2 years of age suffered meningitis (infection of the membranes and fluid that cover the brain and spinal cord); 700 had bacteremia (infection of the bloodstream); 2,200 had pneumonia (infection of the lungs); and 200,000 had an ear infection — all caused by pneumococcal bacteria.

After Vaccine

The current purified polysaccharide vaccine (licensed in Canada in 1983) contains polysaccharides from the 23 strains that cause over 90% of serious infections in adults. The vaccine is used primarily in the elderly (persons aged 65 and over) and in persons with medical conditions that increase the risk of serious pneumococcal infection. In most parts of Canada, the vaccine is used routinely in adults aged 65 and over to protect against death and severe illness due to pneumococcal infection.

The purified polysaccharide vaccine was never used routinely in children. Unfortunately, it is not effective in children less than 2 years of age, the group at highest risk of pneumococcal disease.

Fortunately, a new form of the vaccine has been developed — the conjugate vaccine — that is very effective in children under age 2, especially in infants (children under 12 months of age). It was licensed in Canada in June 2001. It is the first pneumococcal vaccine that can be expected to have a major impact on the frequency of severe pneumococcal infections. At the time of writing, individuals in most provinces and territories must pay for the vaccine.

The Germ

How It Causes Illness

Pneumococcal bacteria infect only humans and can cause a wide range of infections. Infection starts in the nose or throat, where the bacteria attach to the cells lining the surface.

Infection in carriers. Many people do not develop any symptoms of illness after becoming infected with pneumococci (a silent infection). Such people are called carriers. Carriage of pneumococci can begin early in the first year of life and is very common at all ages. It is estimated that 40% of people become carriers of pneumococcal bacteria in their first year of life!

The pneumococci may persist in the nose and throat for weeks to months. The carrier (silent) infection induces a specific immune response against the serotype (strain) causing the infection, but may not produce any protection against other pneumococcal serotypes. So as the body becomes immune to one serotype, a new serotype will silently infect the person, and the process of building immunity to another strain starts again.

Infection in non-carriers. Pneumococcal bacteria have an external coat, called a capsule, which is made of a large, complex sugar or polysaccharide. The capsule protects the bacteria against attack by the white blood cells, the body's main defence against infection. In someone who lacks antibodies to the strain of pneumococcus infecting the nose and throat, the white blood cells are unable to attack and kill the bacteria. Therefore, the bacteria can invade the body, multiply freely and cause disease.

While the capsule protects pneumococcal bacteria from attack by white blood cells, other parts of the wall of the bacteria cause the damage. When materials from the cell wall of the pneumococcus are released into the body, they cause an intense reaction, called inflammation.

How Pneumococci Are Spread

Healthy carriers. Pneumococci are quite common and live in the back of the nose and throat. Up to 40% of people of all ages are healthy carriers of pneumococci. The spread of pneumococci most often involves carriers rather than persons ill with invasive disease. Fortunately, pneumococcal infections are not highly contagious.

Direct contact. Spread from an infected person to another person requires close, direct contact, through activities such as kissing, coughing and sneezing. The bacteria can also be spread through saliva when sharing items such as cigarettes, lipstick, food or drinks (e.g., from cutlery, cups, water bottles, cans, drinking straws), toothbrushes, toys, mouthguards and musical instruments with mouthpieces.

Children who attend childcare centres or in-home daycares have significantly higher carrier rates of pneumococci than do children cared for in their own home because of the greater frequency and level of contact they have with other children.

The Illness

The most common form of pneumococcal infection is the carrier or silent infection in which a person has pneumococci on the surface of the nose and throat, but develops no illness. Typically, carriage of pneumococci begins early in infancy and remains throughout life. Usually one serotype is carried at a time and may persist for several months before the body develops immunity to it. The person usually starts carrying a new serotype soon afterwards. This process continues throughout a carrier's life.

There are **two types of infections produced by pneumococci:**
- local infections of the respiratory tract, which remain on the surface and surrounding tissues;
- invasive infections, involving an infection of the bloodstream that spreads to organs and tissues.

TABLE 13.1

Types of pneumococcal infections

TYPE OF INFECTION	BODY PART INVOLVED	DISEASE
Local	Ear	Acute otitis
	Sinus	Acute sinusitis
	Bronchi or airways	Acute bronchitis
	Lung	Pneumonia
Invasive	Blood	Bacteremia
		Septicemia
	Central nervous system	Meningitis
	Heart	Endocarditis
	Joint	Septic arthritis
	Bone	Osteomyelitis
	Abdominal lining	Peritonitis

Local infections. When a new serotype of pneumococci (one against which a person has no immunity) infects the lining of the nose and throat, there is a high risk of the bacteria causing disease somewhere in the respiratory tract. In young children, illness — usually an ear infection — occurs in about 15% within 1 month of being infected with a new serotype. Often such infections follow a viral infection of the respiratory tract. The damage to the lining cells (caused by the virus) makes it easier for the bacteria to invade and cause more damage.

Ear infections, called acute otitis, are the most common type of illness caused by pneumococci. Acute otitis is the most common reason for infants and young children to receive antibiotics. Very few children escape having at least one attack of acute otitis in the first 5 years of life. About 20% of children have frequent attacks of otitis, that is, three or more attacks per year, and are called otitis-prone children. Pneumococcal bacteria cause 40–60% of all attacks of ear infections and are the most frequent cause of recurrent attacks in the otitis-prone child.

Pneumococci are also the most common cause of *acute sinusitis*. Like otitis, most cases of sinusitis occur as a complication of a viral infection of the nose and throat. Sinusitis is an infection of the sinuses (sinuses are air-filled spaces within the bones of the cheeks, forehead and nose).

These spaces are connected to the nasal space by means of very narrow openings. With a common cold, these openings can become obstructed and bacteria in the nose may spread into the sinuses. The infection causes inflammation and accumulation of pus in the sinuses, resulting in pain, local tenderness and fever.

The most serious infection of the respiratory tract caused by the pneumococcus bacterium is *pneumonia*, an infection involving the alveoli (or air spaces in the lungs where oxygen enters the body and carbon dioxide leaves) in the lungs. Such infection is characterized by fever, rapid respirations (greater than 50 breaths per minute in children less than 2 years old, more than 40 breaths per minute in older children), cough that often produces yellow or greenish sputum, and chest pain.

Most children and adults with pneumococcal pneumonia will have abnormal chest X-rays because of the inflammation and accumulation of fluid and cells in the air spaces of the lung. A small proportion of those with pneumococcal pneumonia (less than 1 in 10) will also have infection of blood (bacteremia) at the same time as the pneumonia.

Invasive infections. Spread of pneumococci from the nose and throat into the blood results in an infection called *bacteremia*. Pneumococcal bacteremia can occur without spread to other organs, especially in children less than 2 years of age. Such infection (which requires treatment) is very difficult to distinguish from a viral infection (which requires no treatment) because in the early stages, the only sign of illness may be high fever. (More than 95% of children younger than age 2 with high fever have a viral infection, not a serious bacterial infection.) High fever by itself is not harmful. But early in the illness, a doctor cannot identify the germ (i.e., bacteria or virus) that is causing the high fever. This difficulty in diagnosis — although unavoidable — can lead to more serious illness.

Septicemia is the much more severe form of bacteremia. The bacteria grow very rapidly in the blood and overwhelm the body. While in the blood, the bacteria release materials from their cell walls. If the concentration of such materials becomes very high, they damage small blood vessels in the skin and the heart, lungs, kidneys and other organs. As a result, the person may develop shock (a drop in blood pressure) and failure of many organs in the body. This form of the illness can kill very rapidly: the total time from the first symptom of fever to death may be as short as 8 to 12 hours.

Such overwhelming infections are rare in otherwise healthy persons. However, children and adults in whom the spleen is either missing (due to surgery or congenital defect) or not able to function normally (because of disease such as sickle-cell disease) are at greatly increased risk of pneumococcal septicemia. The spleen functions as a filter and helps remove bacteria from the blood. In its absence, bacteria can grow very rapidly to high concentrations. Persons with AIDS are also at increased risk of severe pneumococcal infections.

Infection of other body parts. Once pneumococci enter the bloodstream, they can infect almost any other part of the body, such as the lungs, joints, bones, heart and skin.

Meningitis results when the bacteria in the blood spread into the fluid and membranes covering the brain and spinal cord. In meningitis, the blood supply to the brain can be affected by inflammation and obstruction of blood vessels. Since brain cells cannot withstand interruption of their blood supply for very long, inflammation can result in permanent brain damage. The early signs of meningitis can be very similar to those of flu and other viral infections. This makes diagnosis very difficult, especially in infants. The symptoms of meningitis are summarized below.

TABLE 13.2

Symptoms of pneumococcal meningitis

IN OLDER CHILDREN AND ADULTS	IN BABIES
Fever, usually high (greater than 40°C/104°F)	Fever
Drowsiness or impaired consciousness	Difficulty in awakening
Irritability, fussiness, agitation	Fretfulness or irritability, especially when handled
Severe headache	Difficulty feeding
Vomiting	Vomiting
Stiff neck	Stiff neck and bulging of the fontanelle (soft spot on top of skull) may occur in young babies, but usually not early in the illness
Pain on moving neck	n/a

Complications

Pneumococcal disease can be very severe. About 20% of patients (1 out of 5) with **pneumococcal meningitis** die of the disease, even with appropriate treatment. Deafness occurs in 5–10% of survivors of meningitis, and permanent brain damage occurs in an additional 10–15%. **Pneumococcal septicemia** kills 20–40% of patients. **Pneumococcal pneumonia** is a common cause of death in the elderly.

Although **pneumococcal ear infections** do not kill, if the first attack occurs early in the first year of life, there is a high probability of frequent recurrences over the next few years. Such attacks may be complicated by perforation of the eardrum, which, if severe, may require surgery. Rarely, the infection may spread from the ear to the bone surrounding the ear space, causing *acute mastoiditis*, a potentially fatal infection requiring surgical drainage of the infected bone.

Complications of **bacteremia** result when the bacteria in the blood settle in some part of the body, such as a joint (infective arthritis), bone (osteomyelitis) or heart valve (bacterial endocarditis).

Diagnosis

Diagnosis of pneumococcal disease depends on identification of the pneumococcal bacteria in cultures of blood, cerebrospinal fluid, or other infected sites in the body. Diagnosis of meningitis can be confirmed only by performing a lumbar puncture on the patient. A special needle is inserted into the spinal canal in the lower back and a small amount of fluid is removed. The extracted fluid is examined for the presence of bacteria, increased numbers of white blood cells, and changes in the concentrations of protein and sugar.

Treatment

Antibiotics. Before antibiotics became available, pneumococcal meningitis killed 100% of patients. With antibiotic treatment, the death rate has been reduced to about 10%. Antibiotic treatment is given for 7 to 10 days or longer, depending on the severity of the illness.

Delay in diagnosis and treatment of meningitis increases the risk of deafness and brain damage.

Antibiotics do lead to more rapid relief of symptoms in children with ear infections. However, overuse of antibiotics for colds and other minor respiratory infections has led to a great increase in the proportion of bacteria that are resistant to commonly used antibiotics.

Post-recovery. The immunity following a pneumococcal infection corresponds specifically with the serotype (strain) that caused the infection. Therefore, the person should be vaccinated to develop immunity against the other serotypes.

The Vaccine

Types of Vaccines

Purified bacterial polysaccharide. There are two types of pneumococcal vaccines, both of which are made from purified substances extracted from the bacteria. Because the vaccines are highly purified chemicals, not whole bacteria, it is impossible to get the disease from the vaccine. The polysaccharide vaccine is used in older children and adults, while the conjugate vaccine is most suitable for children under age 2.

Pneumococcal polysaccharide vaccine. Bacteria have unique proteins and complex sugars on their surfaces called *antigens*. They are very different from human proteins and sugars. Some surface antigens enable the germ to stick to human cells (this is the first step of infection). Others protect the germ against the body's defences. The immune system targets these bacterial antigens.

The original pneumococcal vaccine is a mixture of highly purified chemicals extracted from 23 serotypes of pneumococci. These "chemicals" are complex sugars (called polysaccharides) that form the capsule or outer coat of the bacteria. The polysaccharides protect the bacteria from being attacked and destroyed by white blood cells. If a person has antibody, the antibodies combine with the polysaccharides and coat the surface of the bacteria, making it very easy for the white blood cells to ingest and kill the bacteria.

Pneumococcal conjugate vaccine. This new pneumococcal vaccine was licensed in Canada in June 2001. Like the *Haemophilus influenzae* type b conjugate vaccine [see Chapter 7] and the new meningococcal conjugate vaccines [see Chapter 14], this new vaccine consists of purified polysaccharides, which are then chemically linked to a purified protein (conjugate means "joined together"). The process of linking the purified sugar to a protein carrier results in a vaccine that is much more effective in young children, including infants.

The 7 pneumococcal serotypes used to make the vaccine were chosen from among the more than 90 possible strains of pneumococci because they are the most common causes of invasive pneumococcal infections in infants and young children in Canada.

How Pneumococcal Vaccines Are Made

Process for pneumococcal polysaccharide vaccine. The vaccine for each of the 23 strains or serotypes of pneumococci is prepared separately. Pneumococcal bacteria are grown in liquid culture. When growth is complete, the bacteria are removed and the polysaccharide is extracted from the fluid and purified. The 23 different polysaccharides used in the purified polysaccharide vaccine are then combined to make the final product.

Process for pneumococcal conjugate vaccine. To make the conjugated vaccine, the purified polysaccharides of the 7 chosen serotypes of pneumococci are prepared and then chemically linked to a protein. The protein, called CRM, is highly purified and is similar to diphtheria toxoid (both diphtheria and tetanus toxoids are proteins).

Additives. The vaccine does *not* contain thimerosal, a mercury-containing preservative.

Testing. Mandatory tests for potency (effectiveness), toxicity and sterility are carried out on all lots (batches) of vaccine before they can be distributed [see Chapter 2, under *Vaccine safety*].

Available Forms of Pneumococcal Vaccine

Combinations. Neither the pure polysaccharide vaccine nor the conjugate vaccine is available combined with any other vaccines. Each must be administered separately.

Vaccines for different age groups. The conjugate vaccine is used for children less than 2 years of age.

Boosters (to enhance prior vaccinations). Booster doses are not routinely recommended for either vaccine.

How the Vaccines Are Given

Both the polysaccharide and the conjugate vaccines are given by intramuscular injection. The polysaccharide vaccine can also be given subcutaneously.

Schedule of Vaccination

Children under age 2. The National Advisory Committee on Immunization recommends routine immunization of all children less than 2 years of age with the new *pneumococcal conjugate vaccine*. The recommended schedule is summarized in Table 13.3, below.

Children ages 2 to 5. In healthy children 24 to 59 months of age, vaccination should be considered (with the conjugate vaccine) because there is a moderate risk of invasive pneumococcal disease in this age group. As well, attendance at group childcare increases the risk of pneumococcal disease. Children attending childcare centres have a greater risk of pneumococcal disease than children cared for in their own home, but all children 2 to 5 years of age are at some risk and therefore would benefit from the vaccine.

Children in this age group who are at increased risk of pneumococcal disease because of a medical condition [see Text Box below] should be vaccinated with 2 doses of conjugate vaccine, at least 8 weeks apart, followed by 1 dose of pneumococcal polysaccharide vaccine given 8 weeks after the second dose of conjugate vaccine. The first 2 doses of conjugate vaccine stimulate immune memory so that the polysaccharide vaccine (used for the third dose) can induce a good antibody response.

TABLE 13.3

Recommended* schedule of vaccination with pneumococcal conjugate vaccine, under age 5

AGE AT FIRST DOSE	PRIMARY SERIES	BOOSTER DOSE
2 to 6 months	3 doses, 8 weeks apart	1 dose at 12 to 15 months of age
7 to 11 months	2 doses, 8 weeks apart	1 dose at 12 to 15 months of age, and at least 4 weeks after the last dose of the primary series.
12 to 23 months	2 doses, 8 weeks apart	None
24 to 59 months	1 dose	None

* *The vaccine is considered part of routine immunization for children aged 2 to 23 months; it is recommended for children aged 24 to 59 months.*

Children age 5 and over and adults. A single dose of *pneumococcal polysaccharide vaccine* is recommended for the following persons because they are at increased risk of severe or fatal pneumococcal infections:

- all persons 65 years of age or older;
- adults and children over 5 years of age whose spleen has been removed or who have sickle-cell disease;
- adults and children over 5 years of age with certain medical conditions, such as those listed in the Text Box [at right].

Duration of protection. The duration of protection after use of the *polysaccharide vaccine* is not known. The **conjugate vaccine** produces a high level of protection against disease caused by the 7 serotypes in the vaccine. Because the conjugate vaccine induces immune memory [see *The results of vaccination*, below], protection is expected to last many years, if not for life.

Possible Side Effects of Pneumococcal Vaccines

The **pneumococcal polysaccharide vaccine** is very safe. Local reactions are rarely severe. Redness, swelling, pain and tenderness

Medical conditions that increase the risk of invasive pneumococcal disease

- Sickle-cell disease and certain other congenital disorders of hemoglobin (part of red blood cells)
- Non-functioning or missing spleen due to disease, congenital defect or surgery
- HIV infection and AIDS
- Chronic heart or lung disease (excluding asthma, other than in children on high-dose corticosteroid treatment)
- Diabetes mellitus (chronic condition of impaired carbohydrate, protein and fat metabolism)
- Cerebrospinal fluid leak
- Conditions that lead to suppression of the immune system, including:
  - cancers such as leukemia, lymphoma, Hodgkin's disease
  - chronic renal (kidney) failure or nephrotic syndrome
  - immunosuppressive chemotherapy, including long-term systemic corticosteroids
  - kidney, liver, heart, lung or bone marrow transplant

occur at the injection site in 15–20% of recipients. Fever and other generalized reactions are uncommon. The vaccine has not been shown to cause any serious adverse events. It can be given at the same time as other childhood vaccines such as DTaP/IPV+Hib, MMR, varicella (chickenpox), and meningococcal C conjugate vaccines.

The **pneumococcal conjugate vaccine** is also very safe. Local reactions (e.g., redness, swelling, soreness) occur in 10–20% of recipients, but the reactions are mild and last only 1 to 2 days. Local reactions, especially redness, are more common after the pneumococcal conjugate vaccine than after DTaP/IPV+Hib conjugate vaccine. Fever, irritability and other general reactions are not increased in frequency or severity by giving pneumococcal conjugate vaccine at the same time as any of the combination vaccines (e.g., DTaP, DTaP/IPV+Hib vaccines). Two conjugate vaccines given at the same time must be injected at two separate sites, however; some may experience local reactions at both injection sites.

Reasons to Avoid or Delay Pneumococcal Vaccines

Do not give. Neither the *polysaccharide* nor the *conjugate vaccine* should be given to persons who are allergic to any component of the vaccine or who have had an allergic reaction (hives; swelling of face, lips or throat; wheezing; and/or shock [fall in blood pressure]) to a previous dose of the vaccine.

For children under the age of 2, the *polysaccharide vaccine* is not recommended because of its ineffectiveness in that age group.

Do not delay. Vaccination should not be deferred or delayed because of minor illnesses, such as the common cold, with or without fever. Such infections do not increase the risk of local reactions and do not interfere with the immune response to vaccination.

Delay. Moderate to severe illness, with or without fever, is a reason to delay routine immunization. This precaution may be taken in order to avoid the possibility of adding any side effects of the vaccine on top of the effects of the illness itself.

The Results of Vaccination

Studies reveal need for vaccine. The first large-scale North American program to attempt to reduce the death rate due to pneumococcal disease was launched in Ontario in 1996 for two reasons: studies in Ontario found that persons of all ages with chronic illness are at increased risk of getting pneumococcal disease [see Text Box above, *Medical conditions that increase the risk of invasive pneumococcal disease*]; and studies in Toronto (1993) found that 7% of strains of pneumococci are resistant to penicillin.

Through the program, the *pneumococcal polysaccharide vaccine* is provided at no cost to the following persons:
• all residents of nursing homes, homes for the aged and chronic care facilities;
• all adults and children over 2 years of age with chronic illnesses;
• all adults aged 65 and over, with or without medical conditions.

Most other Canadian provinces and territories have introduced similar vaccine programs.

Unfortunately, the polysaccharide vaccine is not effective in children less than 2 years of age, the age group with the highest rate of both local and invasive forms of pneumococcal disease. Infants and young children do not make an adequate immune response to the purified polysaccharides.

The *pneumococcal conjugate vaccine* is much more effective than the pneumococcal polysaccharide vaccine in stimulating antibody in people of all ages, including infants as young as 2 months of age. More importantly, unlike the polysaccharide vaccine, the conjugate vaccine also induces immune memory. [See Chapter 1 for a discussion of immune response and immune memory.]

The vaccine will stimulate production of memory T-cells in a person, which enables the immune system to respond very rapidly and protect against a germ it has seen before. If in the future the person encounters any of the 7 serotypes of pneumococci that are in the vaccine — even if the amount of antibody present in the blood has decreased to low or even non-detectable levels — immune memory will kick in and protect against infection. Because the conjugate vaccine induces immune memory, protection is expected to last many years, if not a lifetime.

Evidence that the vaccines work includes the following:
• The *polysaccharide vaccine* is about 80% effective in healthy young adults in preventing disease caused by the 23 serotypes present in the vaccine. It doesn't protect against the pneumococcal

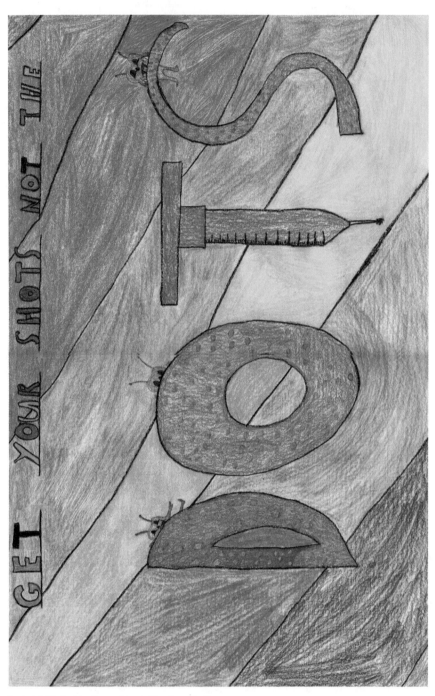

Frederick W. Chubbs, Corner Brook, Newfoundland

serotypes that are not in the vaccine, but 90% of all pneumococcal infections are caused by just 23 serotypes.

- The *polysccharide vaccine* is 50–75% effective in people over the age of 65 (the group at increased risk of dying from pneumococcal infections). At a glance, this rate of protection may not seem great; but it is actually quite good considering that immune responses to vaccines are known to deteriorate with aging.
- A large study, involving almost 40,000 infants in northern California who were vaccinated at 2, 4, 6 and 15 months of age, demonstrated that the *conjugate vaccine* is 97% effective in preventing invasive pneumococcal bacteremia and meningitis in this age group.
- The *conjugate vaccine* has been shown to reduce ear infections and pneumonia in infants: acute otitis with a perforated eardrum was reduced by 65%; and pneumonia with an abnormal chest X-ray was reduced by 33%. Studies in children in childcare centres in Israel have demonstrated similar reductions in otitis and pneumonia. These rates probably don't reflect the true level of protection the vaccine provides against these infections. Because it is difficult to identify the cause of ear infections and pneumonia, the vaccine does not get credit for having an effect on many cases of these "unknown cause" infections.
- The *conjugate vaccine* has also been shown to reduce carriage of the vaccine serotypes by 40–50%. Vaccinated children have the same overall carrier rate of pneumococci compared with unvaccinated children because they can just as easily carry the strains not in the vaccine. Fortunately, the serotypes of pneumococci which are not in the vaccine are much less likely to cause serious disease than the serotypes contained in the vaccine.

Summary

- Both the purified pneumococcal polysaccharide vaccine and the pneumococcal conjugate vaccine are very safe.
- Routine immunization of children less than 2 years old with the new pneumococcal conjugate vaccine is very effective in preventing invasive pneumococcal bacteremia and meningitis.

- Routine immunization of children less than 2 years old with the new pneumococcal conjugate vaccine is effective in reducing acute otitis and pneumonia caused by pneumococci and in reducing the carrier rate of serotypes contained in the vaccine.
- Routine immunization of infants, children and adults at increased risk of invasive pneumococcal disease because of age or underlying medical condition is effective in reducing death and severe disease.

CHAPTER 14

Meningococcal Disease

The bacterium called meningococcus (*Neisseria meningitidis*) causes meningitis, bacteremia, septicemia and other invasive infections. Death from all forms of severe meningococcal disease occurs in about 1 out of 10 cases (10%), even with treatment and intensive care.

Meningitis is an infection of the membranes and fluid that cover the brain and spinal cord. Bacteremia is an infection of the bloodstream, and severe bacteremia is called septicemia. It can progress very rapidly, causing shock (low blood pressure) and damage to many organs in the body. Death from overwhelming shock can occur within 6 to 12 hours after the first sign of illness.

Most spread of the bacteria occurs via healthy carriers in the general population. About 20% of adolescents and adults are healthy carriers of meningococci. Cigarette smoking — both active and passive (inhaling second-hand smoke) — increases the risk of becoming a carrier.

There are 13 different strains or groups of meningococci, which can be distinguished from each other by differences in their outer coating. Groups A, B, C, Y and W135 cause almost all cases of meningococcal disease.

A History of Meningococcal Disease

Before Vaccine

Before 1950, group A strains caused very large epidemics every 7 to 10 years in many parts of the world. In the last such epidemic in Canada, between 1940 and 1943, there were over 2,600 cases per year. Fortunately, there have been no large group A epidemics in Canada, the United States, or other developed nations since the end of World War II.

Very large epidemics of group A disease continue to occur in other parts of the world: almost every year in the "meningitis belt" (sub-Saharan Africa), and at less frequent intervals in China, India and other less developed countries.

Since 1950, group B and group C strains have caused most cases of meningococcal disease in Canada.

After Vaccine

Effective vaccines against groups A and C meningococci were developed by the U.S. army in the late 1960s. Meningococcal outbreaks had always been a problem in the military, especially among recruits during wartime. The group C vaccine was shown to be almost 90% effective in preventing disease in army recruits between 1968 and 1970. Since 1972, military recruits in the United States, Canada and many other countries have been routinely vaccinated upon entry into the forces, and group C outbreaks have disappeared within this population.

Groups A and C vaccines (individually and combined) have been effective in controlling outbreaks both in the general population and among military recruits. Unfortunately, the group C vaccine is not effective in children less than 2 years old, the age group at greatest risk of disease. As well, the protection induced by the original meningococcal vaccines did not last more than 3 to 5 years, so the vaccines were not useful for routine immunization.

New forms of the vaccines became available in Canada in 2001 and have proven to be very effective in people of all ages. These vaccines have now been recommended for routine use in all infants. This is expected to significantly reduce the number of cases of meningococcal disease that occur in Canada every year, which ranges between 200 and 400. At the time of writing, individuals in most provinces and territories must pay for the vaccine.

The Germ

How It Causes Illness

Meningococcal bacteria infect only humans. Infection starts in the nose or throat where the bacteria attach to the cells lining the surface.

Infection in carriers. Many people do not develop any symptoms of illness after becoming infected with meningococci. Such people are called carriers. The meningococci may persist in the nose and throat of carriers for weeks or months.

The carrier, or silent, infection induces a specific immune response against the strain causing the infection, but may not produce any protection against other meningococcal strains. As the body becomes immune to one strain, a new strain can silently infect the person, and the process of building immunity to another strain starts.

Infection in non-carriers. Meningococcal bacteria have an external coat called a capsule. It is made of a large, complex sugar (or polysaccharide).

The capsule protects the bacteria against attack by the body's white blood cells, which are a vital defence against infection. In someone who lacks antibodies to the strain of meningococci infecting the nose and throat, the white blood cells are unable to attack and kill the bacteria. Therefore, the bacteria can invade the body, multiply freely and cause disease.

Endotoxin causes inflammation. While the capsule protects meningococcal bacteria from attack by white blood cells, another part of the wall of the bacteria, called endotoxin, causes the damage. This complex chemical is present in many different bacteria. When endotoxin is released in the body, it causes an intense reaction called inflammation. If the bacterial infection is not treated, the inflammation can get out of control and cause damage throughout the body, especially to blood vessels.

How Meningococci Are Spread

Healthy carriers. Meningococci bacteria are quite common and live in the back of the nose and throat without causing damage or illness. About 20% of adolescents and adults are healthy carriers of meningococci. Carriers may be infected for short periods (weeks) or many months. (Cigarette smoking, both active and passive smoking [inhaling second-hand smoke], increases the risk of becoming a carrier and therefore of spreading the bacteria to others.)

Direct contact. The spread of meningococci most often involves carriers rather than persons ill with invasive disease. Spread from an infected person (carriers included) to another person requires close, direct contact, through such activities as kissing, coughing and sneezing. It can also be spread through saliva when sharing items such as cigarettes, lipstick, food or drinks (e.g., from cutlery, cups, water bottles, cans, drinking straws), toothbrushes, toys, mouthguards and musical instruments with mouthpieces.

Not highly contagious. Fortunately, the bacteria are extremely fragile outside the body; for this reason, meningococcal infections are not highly contagious.

Daily contact. The risk of spread is greatly increased by daily contact. Family members and others living with someone who is ill with meningococcal infection are at increased risk of disease. Although the risk of spread within a household is higher than that in the general public, the risk is still small, reflecting the slow spread of the infection. More than 1 case of meningococcal disease occurs in about 1–3% of families, almost always within 1 to 2 weeks of each other.

The Illness

Carrier state of infection. The most common form of meningococcal infection is the carrier or silent infection in which a person has meningococci on the surface of the nose and throat, but develops no illness. The frequency of the carrier state is very low in infants (children less than 12 months of age) and young children, low in older children, and highest (10–30%) in adolescents and young adults.

A person may remain a carrier of the same strain of meningococcus for a long time — up to 6 months or more. Once immunity to that strain develops, the person is able to get rid of the bacteria. Until a person has developed immunity to all of the strains, they are still considered susceptible to the infection.

Resulting conditions of invasive infection. Invasive meningococcal disease most often results in meningitis or septicemia. About 40% of patients have meningitis alone; 40% have both meningitis and septicemia; 10–15% have septicemia alone; and 5% have other forms of illness such as pneumonia (an infection of the lungs) and infected joints.

Meningitis results when the bacteria in the blood spread into the fluid and membranes covering the brain and spinal cord. In meningitis, the blood supply to the brain can be affected by inflammation and obstruction of blood vessels. Since brain cells cannot withstand interruption of their blood supply for very long, inflammation can result in permanent brain damage.

Septicemia is the most severe form of meningococcal disease. With this type of infection, the bacteria grow very rapidly in the blood and overwhelm the body. While in the blood, the bacteria release endotoxin (poison) from their cell wall. If the concentration of endotoxin becomes very high, it causes damage to small blood vessels in the skin, heart, lungs, kidneys and other organs. As a result, the person may develop shock (fall in blood pressure) and failure of many organs in the body.

This form of the illness can kill very rapidly: the total time from the first symptom of fever to death may be as short as 6 to 12 hours.

Other infections. Once meningococci enter the bloodstream, they can infect almost any other part of the body, such as the lungs, joints, bones, heart and skin.

Symptoms of meningococcal disease. A *characteristic rash* is the single most specific and most noticeable symptom of invasive meningococcal disease. The rash starts as small red spots anywhere on the body. At first, the spots may fade when pressed on, but within an hour or two, they no longer fade. The spots may spread rapidly to all parts of the body. In severe cases, the spots rapidly enlarge in size and may look like large bruises under the skin.

The rash occurs in two-thirds of cases of meningococcal meningitis and in almost all cases of meningococcal septicemia. Sometimes the rash does not develop until the disease is quite advanced. The rash is caused by damage to the small blood vessels in the skin, leading to small areas of bleeding into the skin, which are called petechiae.

In meningitis and septicemia. The early signs of meningococcal meningitis and septicemia can be very similar to those of flu and other viral infections. This makes diagnosis very difficult. The symptoms of meningococcal meningitis and septicemia are summarized in Table 14.1, at right.

It is important to recognize that meningococcal septicemia and meningitis have different symptoms. In particular, septicemia often begins with fever, aches and pains, nausea, loss of appetite, and vague sensations of feeling unwell. The rash usually starts within a few hours of the start of the fever. Septicemia usually lacks the typical symptoms of meningitis such as severe headache, stiff neck, or pain on flexing the neck and back.

TABLE 14.1

Symptoms of meningococcal meningitis and septicemia

SYMPTOM	MENINGITIS	SEPTICEMIA
Fever, usually high (40°C/104°F or more)	X	X
Drowsiness/impaired consciousness	X	X
Irritability, fussiness, agitation	X	X
Severe headache	X	
Vomiting	X	X
Stiff neck	X	
Pain on moving neck	X	
Rash	X – not always	X
Cold hands and feet		X
Rapid breathing		X
Pain in muscles, joints, abdomen		X

In babies less than 1 year of age, meningitis may be more difficult to identify because specific symptoms (e.g., stiff neck, bulging soft spot on the skull) usually do not occur right away.

Infection in other body parts. Symptoms of infection in other parts of the body are specific to the part affected. For example, with arthritis, there is pain in the joint or bone.

Symptoms of meningococcal meningitis in infants

- Fever
- Fretfulness or irritability, especially when handled
- Difficulty in awakening
- Difficulty feeding
- Vomiting
- Stiff neck and bulging of the fontanelle (soft spot on top of the skull)

Complications

Meningococcal disease can be very severe and progress very rapidly. Overall, about 1 patient in 10 (10%) dies in spite of prompt diagnosis and appropriate treatment. Deafness occurs in 1–2% of survivors of meningitis. Permanent brain damage is uncommon.

Meningococcal septicemia kills 20–40% of patients; meningitis kills about 5%. A study of the outcomes of a group C outbreak in Quebec in the early 1990s revealed the following:

- 10% of patients with meningococcal septicemia had scars at areas where gangrene of the skin developed;
- 5% had amputations of one or more extremity;
- 1% had kidney damage.

Diagnosis

Identifying the rash. Unlike rashes due to allergy or to viral infections, the meningococcal rash does not fade under pressure. When the side of a glass or tumbler is pressed against the rash and the rash is examined through the glass, it remains visible (known as the "tumbler test"). Most other rashes caused by viruses or allergies will fade under pressure. In early stages when the rash first appears, it may fade under pressure, but as it develops (within a few hours) it will no longer fade. The "tumbler test" should be done hourly to monitor a child who is ill and has a rash.

Cultures and tests. Diagnosis of meningococcal disease depends on identification of the meningococcal bacteria in cultures of blood or cerebrospinal fluid, and even in cultures of the skin rash. A new laboratory test that is more sensitive than culture in identifying meningococcal infections is becoming increasingly available. The test, called PCR, identifies genetic material in the DNA of the bacteria.

Treatment

Antibiotics. Before antibiotics became available, meningococcal meningitis and septicemia killed almost 100% of patients. With antibiotic treatment, the death rate has been reduced to about 10%.

Antibiotic treatment is given for a minimum of 5 days for meningitis and usually 7 to 10 days or longer for septicemia.

New treatment for septicemia. Patients with septicemia almost always require treatment in an intensive care unit because of the severity of the illness. A new form of treatment (still an oral medication) includes a compound called Activated Protein C; it has been successful in reducing the death rate from septicemia.

Post-recovery. Immunity that develops after infection is directed mainly against the particular strain that caused disease. Therefore, vaccination after recovery from any form of meningococcal infection is advised.

The Vaccine

Types of Vaccines

Purified bacterial polysaccharide. There are two types of meningococcal vaccines, both of which are made from purified substances extracted from the bacteria. Because the vaccines are highly purified chemicals, not intact bacteria, it is impossible to get the disease from the vaccine. The polysaccharide vaccine is used in older children and adults, while the conjugate vaccine is most suitable for children under age 2.

Meningococcal polysaccharide vaccines. Bacteria have unique proteins and complex sugars on their surfaces called *antigens*. They are very different from human proteins and sugars. Some surface antigens allow the germ to stick to human cells (this is the first step of infection). Others protect the germ against the body's defences. The immune system targets these bacterial antigens.

The original meningococcal vaccine is a mixture of highly purified chemicals extracted from four strains of meningococci: groups A, C, Y and W135. These "chemicals" are complex sugars (called polysaccharides) that form the capsule or outer coat of the bacteria.

The polysaccharides protect the bacteria from being attacked and destroyed by white blood cells. If a person has antibody, the antibodies combine with the polysaccharides and coat the surface of the bacteria, making it very easy for the white blood cells to ingest and kill the bacteria.

Two meningococcal polysaccharide vaccines are available in Canada: one contains polysaccharides against A and C meningococci; the other contains polysaccharides against A, C, Y and W135 strains.

Meningococcal conjugate vaccines. Two new group C meningococcal vaccines were licensed in Canada in 2001. Like the *Haemophilus influenzae* type b conjugate vaccine [see Chapter 7] and the new pneumococcal conjugate vaccine [see Chapter 13], these new conjugate (meaning "joined together") vaccines consist of the purified group C polysaccharide, which is then chemically linked to a purified protein. The process of linking the purified sugar to a protein carrier results in vaccines that are effective in young infants. These vaccines are called meningococcal C conjugate vaccines.

No vaccine for group B strains. Unfortunately no vaccine is available against group B strains. The group B polysaccharide has been purified, and a vaccine was made and tested, but it did not stimulate an immune response. Groups B and C cause almost all cases of meningococcal disease in Canada. The frequency of group B strains does not vary much from year to year. However, the rate of group C strains peaks every 7 to 10 years, during which time illness due to group C becomes more common than that due to group B.

Group B causes disease mainly in children less than 5 years old, whereas group C affects people aged 10 to 25. Group B strains are less likely to cause septicemia than group C meningococci.

How Meningococcal Vaccines Are Made

Process for meningococcal polysaccharide vaccine. The vaccine for each strain of meningococcus is prepared separately. Meningococcal bacteria are grown in liquid culture. When growth is complete, the bacteria are removed and the polysaccharide is extracted from the fluid and purified. The different polysaccharides are then combined to make the final product.

Process for meningococcal conjugate vaccine. To make the meningococcal C conjugate vaccine, the purified polysaccharide is prepared, as above, and then is chemically linked to a protein. The combined polysaccharide–protein vaccine, known as a *conjugate vaccine*, is very effective in young infants.

Additives. The vaccine does *not* contain thimerosal, a mercury-containing preservative.

Testing. Mandatory tests for potency (effectiveness), toxicity and sterility are carried out on all lots (batches) of vaccine before they can be distributed [see Chapter 2].

Available Forms of Meningococcal Vaccine

Combinations. The meningococcal polysaccharide vaccine is available in two forms: one contains A and C polysaccharides and another contains A, C, Y and W135 polysaccharides. These polysaccharide vaccines and the meningococcal C conjugate vaccine are not available in combination with any other vaccine.

Vaccines for different age groups. The conjugate vaccine is used for children less than 2 years of age.

Boosters (to enhance prior vaccinations). Booster doses of the meningococcal polysaccharide vaccines and meningococcal C conjugate vaccine are not routinely recommended.

How the Vaccines Are Given

Both types of vaccine are given by injection. The polysaccharide vaccines are given subcutaneously and the conjugate vaccine is given intramuscularly.

Schedules of Vaccination

Meningococcal polysaccharide vaccine. See the Text Box for a list of the people who are recommended to receive the polysaccharide vaccines.

Who should receive the polysaccharide vaccines?

- The population at risk during outbreaks of group A or group C disease
- Groups at increased risk of disease, such as military recruits
- Travellers to regions experiencing epidemics
- Adults and children over 2 years old with disease of the spleen, or whose spleen has been removed
- First-year university students [see explanation below]

First-year university students. In the United States, a number of outbreaks of group C meningococcal disease have occurred among university students. Almost all of the outbreaks involved first-year students residing in dormitories or other student residences. It has therefore been recommended that the polysaccharide vaccine be considered for use in first-year university students, especially those who plan to live in dormitories.

Not the best option for children. Although the meningococcal polysaccharide vaccines are safe and have worked well in controlling outbreaks and epidemics of meningococcal disease, they are not recommended for routine use in children for a number of reasons:

- Protection against disease lasts only 3 to 5 years after vaccination.
- A vaccine that provides protection against group B strains is not available (group B causes disease mainly in children less than 5 years old).
- The group C polysaccharide vaccine is not effective in children less than 2 years of age.

Meningococcal C conjugate vaccine. The National Advisory Committee on Immunization [See Chapter 2, under *Making recommendations on vaccine use*] recommended in October 2001 that all Canadian infants should be vaccinated with the new meningococcal C conjugate vaccine. The following schedule has been recommended until routine vaccination of infants is established and all groups at risk have been vaccinated.

- All infants at 2, 4 and 6 months of age (3 doses) should receive the conjugate vaccine at the same time as the DTaP/IPV + Hib vaccine.
- Infants 4 to 11 months of age who have not yet received the vaccine should be given 2 doses, with at least 4 weeks between each dose.
- Children 1 to 4 years of age, adolescents and young adults who have not yet received the vaccine should receive a single dose (the same dose is used in all age groups).
- Children aged 5 to 11 may also receive a single dose of the vaccine. (Children in this age group are at lower risk than others, and therefore are a lower priority for receiving the vaccine.)

Duration of protection. Protection after vaccination with the *polysaccharide vaccine* lasts approximately 3 to 5 years. The relatively short duration of protection reflects the failure of the polysaccharide vaccine to stimulate immune memory. For this reason, the vaccine is not recommended for routine use in the general population.

Protection following immunization with the **meningococcal C conjugate vaccine** lasts many years because the conjugate vaccine induces immune memory.

Who should receive the conjugate vaccine?*

- Infants
- Children ages 1 to 4
- Adolescents
- Young adults
- Children ages 5 to 11 (lower priority)

* Once routine vaccination is established, only infants will require the vaccine.

Possible Side Effects of Meningococcal Vaccines

The **meningococcal polysaccharide vaccines** are very safe. Local redness, swelling, pain and tenderness occur at the injection site in 15–20% of recipients; these local reactions are rarely severe. Fever and other generalized reactions are uncommon.

The polysaccharide vaccines have been given to millions of military recruits in the U.S. and Canadian forces. They have also been given to several million Canadian children in Quebec, Ontario, British Columbia, Alberta and other provinces to control outbreaks of group C disease. The vaccines have not been shown to cause any serious adverse events.

The **meningococcal conjugate vaccines** are also very safe. They have been given to several million children in England, Wales and Ireland during mass vaccination campaigns to stop outbreaks of group C disease.

Since August 2001, more than 1.5 million children have been vaccinated in Quebec and Alberta. The Canadian experience has been identical to that in the United Kingdom and Ireland. Local reactions occur in 10–20% of recipients, but the reactions are mild and last only 1 to 2 days.

Fever, irritability and other general reactions are not increased in frequency or severity by giving meningococcal conjugate vaccine at the same time as any of the combination vaccines (e.g., DTaP, DTaP+Hib vaccines). Two conjugate vaccines given at the same time must be injected at two separate sites, however; some may experience local reaction at both injection sites.

Reasons to Avoid or Delay Meningococcal, Vaccines

Do not give. Neither the *purified polysaccharide* nor the new *polysaccharide conjugate vaccine* should be given to persons who are allergic to any component of the vaccine or to persons who have had an allergic reaction (hives; swelling of face, lips or throat; wheezing; and/or shock [fall in blood pressure]) to a previous dose of the vaccine.

For children under the age of 2, the *polysaccharide vaccine* is not recommended because of its ineffectiveness in that age group.

Do not delay. Vaccination should not be deferred or delayed because of minor illnesses, such as the common cold, with or without fever. Such infections do not increase the risk of local reactions or other side effects and do not interfere with the immune response to vaccination.

Delay. Moderate to severe illness, with or without fever, is a reason to delay routine immunization. This precaution may be taken in order to avoid the possibility of adding any side effects of the vaccine on top of the effects of the illness itself. However, if meningococcal infections are occurring in the community, vaccination is recommended because the risk of this type of infection in an unimmunized child is much greater than the risk of any local reactions.

The Results of Vaccination

Polysaccharide vaccines. The group A and C polysaccharide vaccines have been about 90% effective in preventing disease caused by these strains.
- The group A vaccine is effective in infants as well as in older children and adults.
- The group C vaccine is much less effective in children under 2 years of age than in older children and adults. (The separate vaccines for A and C are not readily available in Canada, but have been used in Africa and other parts of the world.)

The group Y and W135 vaccines induce good antibody responses, but it is not yet known how effective they are in preventing disease. (Assessment of the effectiveness of the Y and W135 vaccines is difficult because disease due to these strains is uncommon.)

Conjugate vaccines. The meningococcal conjugate C vaccines are much more effective than the pure polysaccharide vaccines in stimulating antibody at all ages, including in infants as young as 2 months old. More importantly, unlike the polysaccharide vaccine, the conjugate C vaccine also induces immune memory. [See Chapter 1 for a discussion of immune response and immune memory.]

The vaccine will stimulate production of memory T-cells in a person, which enables the immune system to respond very rapidly and protect against a germ it has seen before. If in the future the person encounters the group C meningococci — even if the amount of antibody present in the blood has decreased to low or even non-detectable levels — immune memory will kick in and protect against infection. Because the conjugate vaccine induces immune memory, protection is expected to last many years, if not a lifetime.

Evidence that meningococcal vaccines work includes:
- a high rate of success against group C strains. The meningococcal conjugate vaccine produces a high level of protection against group C disease. Within 9 months of starting routine vaccination of infants and children in England and Wales (in November 1990), the frequency of group C disease decreased by more than 97% in vaccinated adolescents and by more than 92% in vaccinated infants and toddlers.
- recommendation for routine vaccination of infants by Canada's authority on the subject. After reviewing the research and evidence of studies and testing on the vaccine, the National Advisory Committee on Immunization recommended in October 2001 that all Canadian infants should be vaccinated with the new meningococcal conjugate vaccine.

No vaccine for group B strain. Neither the meningococcal polysaccharide nor conjugate vaccines protect against disease caused by group B meningococci. These vaccines protect against the specific strain types present in the vaccine, and even then, protection is not 100%.

Strains B and C cause 80–90% of cases in Canada. The current vaccines prevent only 30–60% of meningococcal disease. So complete control of meningococcal disease depends on the success of current research aimed at the development of a vaccine that will stimulate immunity against group B meningococci.

Summary

- Both the meningococcal polysaccharide and conjugate vaccines are very safe.
- Immunization with purified polysaccharide meningococcal vaccines has been very effective in controlling outbreaks of group A and group C diseases.
- Routine immunization of infants, children and adolescents with the new meningococcal conjugate vaccines is very effective in preventing group C disease in young people.
- Routine immunization of all military recruits with meningococcal polysaccharide vaccine has eliminated outbreaks of group C disease among this group.
- Complete control of meningococcal disease will not be achieved until an effective vaccine against group B strains is developed.

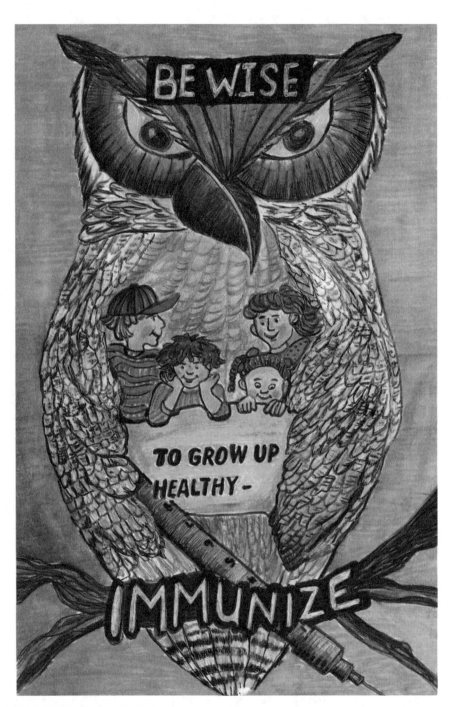

Jasmine Wright, Blind River, Ontario

CHAPTER 15

Chickenpox

Chickenpox (also known as varicella) is an infection caused by varicella-zoster virus (VZ virus). VZ virus also causes zoster (commonly known as shingles). Chickenpox occurs after the first infection with VZ virus. Zoster occurs years or decades after the first infection.

Chickenpox (varicella) is an illness with fever, headache, aches and pains, and a very typical rash that is usually very itchy. The infection is highly contagious. Most cases of chickenpox occur in children under 15 years old. The illness is more severe in teenagers and adults than in children. Some people never get chickenpox in childhood; if exposed to the virus as adults, these people will develop chickenpox, not shingles. First infections with the virus are known as chickenpox, regardless of the age at which the person becomes infected.

Shingles (zoster) is caused by reactivation of the VZ virus, which has persisted in latent or inactive form in certain nerve cells. Zoster is characterized by a localized rash, which may be very itchy and painful. The major complication of zoster is chronic pain at the site of the rash.

Why chickenpox vaccine is needed. Although chickenpox is often a mild disease, it is a costly one, even without complications. Parents generally stay home for an average of 3 days with a child because of chickenpox. The vaccine is cost-effective compared with the wages lost by parents and/or sick-leave benefits incurred by them, the costs of doctor visits and management of the complications of chickenpox. Moreover, chickenpox can lead to complications requiring hospitalization and, in rare cases, to death.

Varicella vaccine is often referred to as the chickenpox vaccine. Both terms are used interchangeably in this book.

A History of Chickenpox

Before Vaccine

Before the varicella vaccine became available, 95% of Canadians would be infected with VZ virus during their lifetime. This means that over 300,000 cases occurred per year.

Over 90% of all cases of chickenpox occur in children less than 15 years of age. Many cases, especially in young children, are mild — so mild that parents may not be aware of the illness. The highest rate of chickenpox occurs in children 5 to 9 years of age, followed closely by children 1 to 4 years of age. This illness occurs throughout the year, but the frequency of cases increases after school opens in September, peaking in the spring and dropping sharply during the summer.

Chickenpox is a mild to moderate illness in the majority of children; itchiness from the rash causes the greatest distress. However, chickenpox or its complications can be severe. Before the vaccine was available, chickenpox resulted in approximately 1,000 hospitalizations and 10 deaths every year in Canada.

After Vaccine

The chickenpox vaccine was licensed in Canada in 1998. In most parts of Canada, parents must purchase the vaccine as it has not yet been included in the routine childhood vaccination programs. Too few children have received the vaccine to be able to detect an effect on the number of cases in Canada.

In the United States, however, the vaccine has been available since 1995. Many states now require proof of vaccination against chickenpox before children may attend school. Between 1972 and 1994, an annual average of 175,837 cases of chickenpox were reported in the U.S. By 1999, only 46,000 cases were reported, a decrease of 73.8%.

Reason for vaccine. Chickenpox is considered by most to be a mild childhood disease. However, the disease bears a significant cost — both health-related and financial. Complications can result from chickenpox and zoster (pneumonia, encephalitis and cerebellar ataxia), some of which can lead to death. [See *Complications*, below, for more information.]

Apart from the health-risk factors, there is a high price tag associated with the illness itself, even for uncomplicated cases: the costs of visits to doctors, medications; days lost from school or paid childcare, and the time and salary lost by parents who stay home to care for the sick child. A recent study in Canada estimated that each case of chickenpox costs $353. A significant 81% of costs were parents' personal expenses and lost salary; only 19% of the costs were incurred by the health care system.

In Canada, 30–65% of children with chickenpox are seen by a doctor. The annual rate of visits to physicians because of chickenpox and zoster varies with the age of the patient, with the peak for chickenpox being in children aged 5 and under and the peak for zoster being in the elderly [see Table 15.1, below].

TABLE 15.1

Physician visits related to chickenpox and zoster, by age of patient

AGE GROUP OF PATIENTS (years)	ANNUAL RATE OF PHYSICIAN OFFICE VISITS RELATED TO ... (per 100 persons)	
	Chickenpox	Zoster
0–4	2.350	0.06
5–14	1.310	0.12
15–44	0.120	0.21
45–64	0.015	0.42
65 and over	0.012	0.77

The Germ

Varicella-zoster (VZ) virus is a member of the herpes family of viruses, which includes the viruses that cause cold sores and genital herpes (herpes simplex), infectious mononucleosis (EB virus), cytomegalovirus disease and roseola (human herpes virus 6). All of these viruses share the following features:

• They are large viruses (large in size compared with most other viruses infecting humans, because they have a complex structure).
• They contain DNA.
• They cause latent (or silent) infection that persists for life.

During the first infection, in addition to causing the rash and other symptoms of chickenpox, VZ virus establishes a silent or latent infection in nerve cells of the dorsal root ganglia, which are collections of specialized nerve cells next to the spinal cord. The viral DNA is incorporated into the human DNA of these nerve cells. During this latent or silent phase of infection, there are no symptoms or other evidence of the presence of VZ virus in the body. The virus does not multiply, although some copying of viral genes occurs.

Reinfections (i.e., a completely new, second infection) with VZ virus do occur, but most produce no illness and can be detected only by special laboratory tests. Rarely do they result in a second attack of chickenpox.

Reactivation. Later in life (usually years later, but highly variable), the VZ virus (which remains in a person for life) in the nerve cells can reactivate, multiply again and spread down the nerve fibres to the skin.

Reactivation results in shingles (also known as zoster), a rash consisting of lesions similar in appearance to those of chickenpox, but which are localized to a relatively small area of skin. The rash is often very itchy and may also be painful. Reactivation is thought to occur as a result of waning immunity to VZ virus, due to either aging or suppression of normal immune function (through disease, such as cancer, or by treatment with medicines that suppress the immune system).

Approximately 10–15% of those infected with VZ virus will develop zoster. The frequency of zoster increases as the interval after chickenpox gets longer. Most cases occur in the elderly.

How It Causes Illness

Chickenpox. When droplets containing chickenpox virus are breathed in, the virus first infects the cells lining the nose and throat. It then spreads to the lymph glands in the neck. After multiplying there for 2 to 3 days, the virus enters the blood (4 to 6 days after infection) and is carried throughout the body to other lymph glands, the liver, spleen and bone marrow where it grows for another 3 to 5 days. The virus then re-invades the blood and spreads to the skin, eyes, respiratory tract and other organs.

The amount of virus in the blood reaches a peak about 11 to 14 days after exposure and then declines rapidly over a few days. The second phase of viremia, or virus present in the blood, coincides with the appearance of the chickenpox rash.

Zoster or shingles results from reactivation of the latent VZ virus in nerve cells; the virus then spreads to the skin. The rash is similar to that of chickenpox, but is localized to the area of skin supplied by the nerves that contain infected nerve cells.

How VZ Virus Is Spread

Highly contagious. *Chickenpox* is highly contagious. The infection spreads very easily from person to person, primarily by exposure to droplets of respiratory secretions containing the virus. The virus can also spread via the rash in two ways: the skin lesions (pox) can release virus into the air; and contamination can occur by touching the lesions.

Children are most contagious the day before the rash appears. (This helps explain the ease of spread.) Contagiousness decreases rapidly after onset of the rash. Children are usually considered contagious for a minimum of 5 days after the rash appears and until all the pox have crusted. [See the Text Box below for the Canadian Paediatric Society's recommendations on attending school or daycare with chickenpox.]

In a household, chickenpox will spread to 60–85% of susceptible persons. The rate of spread of chickenpox is much higher in the household setting than in childcare centres, home care environments or schools.

Patients with *zoster* are also contagious. Susceptible persons acquire chickenpox most often by direct contact with the zoster rash. Very rarely, the virus may spread through the air to a susceptible person.

Attending school or daycare with chickenpox

Because children are most contagious 1 day before to 1 day after the start of the rash, excluding children from daycare centres or from school does little or nothing to stop the spread of chickenpox. By the time the rash appears, the child has already exposed many others to the virus.

For this reason, the Canadian Paediatric Society (CPS) has recommended the discontinuation of the policy of excluding children from daycare or school for 5 days after the start of the rash or until all lesions have crusted. The CPS recommends that children with chickenpox be allowed to return to daycare or school as soon as they feel well enough to participate without requiring extra care, regardless of the number of days since the start of the rash.

The Illness

Chickenpox (Varicella)

Symptoms in children *(pre-rash)*. Following an incubation period of 10 to 21 days (average 14 to 16 days), there may be a short period (1 to 2 days) of fever of 39–40°C (102–104°F) and aches and pains. Most children also have loss of appetite and headache during the first few days of the illness, but none of the symptoms are usually severe.

Rash. In many children, the first sign of illness is the rash. It first appears on the scalp and face and spreads rapidly down the body and onto the arms and legs. The rash is more intense on the face and trunk than on the extremities.

Each skin lesion progresses rapidly from one stage to the next:
- red spot;
- vesicle (a small blister filled with clear fluid);
- pustule (a blister filled with cloudy fluid);
- crust or scab.

New pox appear in crops for up to 3 to 4 days so that lesions in all stages may be present at the same time. The rash is associated with itchiness, which may be very intense and cause great distress to the child.

Symptoms in adults. Chickenpox is much more severe in adults than in children. The rash is more extensive and fever is more common [see below].

TABLE 15.2

Uncomplicated chickenpox in children, adolescents and adults

AGE OF PATIENT (years)	AVERAGE NUMBER OF DAYS DURING WHICH NEW POX CONTINUE TO APPEAR	AVERAGE NUMBER OF POX	PERCENTAGE THAT EXPERIENCE FEVER
2–12	3.4	347	67
13–18	3.2	421	62
Over 18	3.9	500+	90

Shingles (Zoster)

Reactivation of virus. Following primary infection causing chickenpox, VZ virus migrates to nerve cells adjacent to the spinal cord and remains latent. Years later, as a result of waning immunity due to aging, depression of the immune system caused by disease (AIDS, cancer, leukemia, lymphoma) or treatment (cancer chemotherapy, high-dose steroids), VZ virus reactivates, begins to multiply and spreads down a nerve to the skin.

Symptoms. A rash develops on a localized area of skin on one side of the body. Pain, itching or burning may sometimes precede the appearance of the rash. The rash is similar to that of chickenpox, except it is more limited in distribution. The rash is almost always very itchy and is often very painful. It lasts 10 to 15 days without treatment.

Complications

Chickenpox causes an average of 5.8 deaths per year in Canada, with a range of 1 to 16 deaths (children and adults) per year since 1973. The death rate in children is 1 to 3 per 100,000 cases. Over 90% of the deaths occur in previously healthy persons.

The risk of requiring hospitalization because of VZ virus varies with age [see Table below].

TABLE 15.3

Hospitalization from chickenpox and zoster, by age

AGE OF PATIENT (years)	CASES HOSPITALIZED (%)	AVERAGE LENGTH OF HOSPITAL STAY (days)
0–1	1.8	5.5
2–4	0.4	5.0
5–11	0.2	4.5
12–18	0.4	4.6
19–24	0.5	4.3
25–44	1.4	8.7
45–64	1.9	10.2
65 and over	7.0	18.0

Of chickenpox in children. Complications occur in 5–10% of previously healthy children with chickenpox. The most common complications are *pneumonia* (infection of the lungs), *encephalitis* (intense inflamation of the brain; 1 in 5,000 cases) and *cerebellar ataxia* (1 in 4,000 cases). Cerebellar ataxia is the result of inflammation of part of the brain called the cerebellum; it manifests as sudden onset of loss of muscle co-ordination so that the child has difficulty walking and performing voluntary movements.

Flesh-eating disease. More than half of the complications are skin infections resulting from scratching of the itchy rash. While most such skin infections are mild, chickenpox is one of the most common pre-disposing factors for the development of the life-threatening infection called necrotizing fasciitis (or "flesh-eating disease") caused by group A *Streptococcus*.

Other bacterial infections that may complicate chickenpox are uncommon. They include bacteremia (infection of the blood), osteomyelitis (bone infections), joint infections and conjunctivitis (inflammation of the eyelid).

TABLE 15.4

Complications of chickenpox, by group affected

COMPLICATION	GROUP AFFECTED
Bacterial infection of pox	Children
Flesh-eating disease	
Bacteremia, bone and joint infections	
Cerebellar ataxia	
Pneumonia	Adults much more often than children
Encephalitis	
Death	

Of chickenpox in adults. Complications of chickenpox are much more frequent and severe in adults. The death rate from chickenpox is approximately 25 times higher in adults than in children. Only 5% of all chickenpox cases occur in adults, but 55–60% of all deaths due to chickenpox are in adults. The main causes of death in adults with chickenpox are encephalitis and pneumonia.

Of chickenpox during pregnancy. If a woman gets chickenpox during the first 20 weeks of pregnancy, there is a risk that the virus will infect the fetus. Such infection may result in severe damage to the fetus (outlined in Table below), known as congenital varicella syndrome.

TABLE 15.5

Rate of occurrence of features of congenital varicella syndrome in babies whose mothers have had chickenpox during pregnancy

FEATURE	FREQUENCY (%)
Skin scars	70
Blindness or damaged eyes	66
Low birth weight	50
Abnormal growth of extremities	50
Brain damage	45
Death before 14 months of age	28

The risk of congenital varicella syndrome varies with the time of infection during pregnancy. The risk is 0.4% if chickenpox occurs in the first trimester (0 to 12 weeks of pregnancy) and 2.0% for the second trimester (13 to 20 weeks of gestation). The syndrome is very rare if infection occurs after the 20th week.

However, if the mother develops chickenpox around the time of delivery (from 5 days before to 2 days after birth), up to 30% of newborn infants develop very severe chickenpox, with involvement of the brain, heart and liver. About 1 in 5 infected newborns dies.

Of chickenpox in persons with suppressed immune systems. Before the availability of current treatment (specific immune globulin to prevent chickenpox combined with medication to treat chickenpox), children with suppressed immune systems were at high risk for severe chickenpox and death. Children with leukemia, lymphoma, bone marrow and organ transplants, and those on medications that suppress the immune system were included in this high-risk group. However, with current treatment, death has become rare in such children.

Of zoster (shingles). In a small proportion of patients, the shingles rash may spread over the entire body. If zoster involves the eyelids, the cornea may become infected, leading to scarring and possibly blindness.

The most frequent and debilitating complication of zoster is a condition called *postherpetic neuralgia* (constant or intermittent pain that occurs in the area of skin affected by the zoster rash after the rash has disappeared). The pain, which may be severe and incapacitating, may last 3 months or more. Although uncommon after zoster in children or young adults, this condition occurs in over 25% of those who get zoster after age 50.

Diagnosis

The rash of chickenpox is very characteristic and can usually be diagnosed without laboratory tests. A variety of tests are available to detect the virus in skin lesions and antibody responses in blood.

Treatment

Antiviral drugs not recommended for routine use. Both chickenpox and zoster can be treated with a variety of medicines, including acyclovir, valacyclovir, and famcyclovir, either by mouth or intravenously (through an intravenous [IV], drip administered in the hospital). However, these antiviral drugs must be used within 24 hours of the appearance of the chickenpox rash in order to shorten the duration of the illness. The reason antiviral drugs must be started in this very limited time period is that the virus stops multiplying within 72 hours of onset of the rash in persons with normal immune responses. Therefore, antiviral treatment is not recommended for routine use in otherwise healthy children with chickenpox.

Acyclovir and similar antiviral drugs are effective in shortening the duration of the rash in zoster, if started within the first 5 days after onset of the rash. The drugs are not of any benefit in treating postherpetic neuralgia.

Treatment for persons at increased risk. Oral acyclovir should be considered for use in persons at increased risk of severe disease because of age or underlying illness, including otherwise healthy adolescents and adults, those with chronic skin or lung disorders, those on long-term aspirin therapy and those receiving corticosteroids. Treatment is also recommended for those with conditions resulting in suppression of the immune system.

Treatment for those at high risk. Those who are at high risk of severe disease [see Text Box, below] should be protected following exposure to chickenpox by administration of a special preparation of immune globulin known as varicella-zoster immune globulin (VZIG). VZIG contains a high concentration of antibody against varicella virus. For maximum effect, VZIG should be given as soon as possible after exposure to chickenpox. It has little effect if given more than 96 hours after exposure.

Persons at high risk of severe disease after exposure to chickenpox

- Immunocompromised children without a history of chickenpox, including those with HIV infection
- Immunocompromised adolescents and adults known to be susceptible to chickenpox
- Susceptible pregnant women
- Newborn infants whose mothers developed chickenpox within 5 days before and 2 days after delivery
- Hospitalized premature infants whose gestational age was equal to or greater than 28 weeks and whose mothers lack a history of chickenpox
- Hospitalized premature infants whose gestational age was less than 28 weeks or whose birth weight was less than 1000 g, regardless of their mother's history of chickenpox

---

The Vaccine

Type of Vaccine

Chickenpox (varicella) vaccine is a **live attenuated (weakened) virus**. It was licensed in the United States in 1995 and in Canada in December 1998.

Dr. Takahashi in Japan developed chickenpox vaccine from a strain of virus isolated from a 3-year-old boy with chickenpox, named K. Oka. The Oka strain was grown and attenuated in a process involving both human tissue culture cells and guinea pig cells. The current vaccine is derived from the Oka strain and is produced only in human tissue culture cells, named MRC-5 cells. It takes 10 months to produce each lot of vaccine.

How Varicella Vaccine Is Made

Process. After the Oka strain of varicella virus has been grown in human MRC-5 cells, the infected cells are suspended in liquid and broken apart to release the virus. The virus is separated from the cellular waste. The vaccine is then freeze-dried in order to preserve the live virus during transportation and storage. The vaccine is stable for 18 months when stored in a frost-free freezer at −15°C (+5°F) or less.

Additives. Each dose of vaccine contains sucrose (25 mg), sodium chloride (3.2 mg), sodium glutamate (0.5 mg), sodium phosphate dibasic (45 mg), sodium phosphate monobasic (0.08 mg), hydrolyzed gelatin (12.5 mg), trace amounts of EDTA (ethylenediaminetetraacetic acid, a chemical to bind and remove other chemicals during purification), neomycin (an antibiotic) and calf serum. (Calf serum is necessary for proper growth of cells in the test tube.) [See Question 17 in Chapter 17 for more information about calf serum.] The various additives are used to maintain the required acidity during the freeze-drying process and to maintain the "shelf-life" of the virus during storage.

During purification of the vaccine, *all* calf serum and *all* cells (animal and human) are removed. The vaccine does *not* contain thimerosal, a mercury-containing preservative, or any other preservative.

Testing. Tests for potency (effectiveness), toxicity and sterility are carried out on all batches of vaccine, both by the manufacturer and the Bureau of Biologics and Radiopharmaceuticals. [See Chapter 2 for more detail.]

Available Forms of Varicella Vaccine

Combinations. The varicella vaccine is not yet available in combination with any other vaccines. Research to combine it with the measles, mumps and rubella (MMR) vaccine is underway.

Vaccines for older children and adults. The same dosage of vaccine is used for all age groups.

Boosters (to enhance prior vaccinations). At this time, boosters are not necessary.

How the Vaccine Is Given

The vaccine is supplied in single-dose vials containing the freeze-dried powder. The powder is mixed with a precise amount of sterile water immediately before use. The vaccine is given by injection under the skin (subcutaneously).

Schedule of Vaccination

Children. The vaccine should be given after the first birthday. Children 1 to 12 years of age should receive 1 dose of vaccine.

Varicella vaccine may be given with MMR vaccine, DTaP/IPV+Hib vaccine or DTaP/IPV, at separate sites with separate syringes, at a single office visit. If not given at the same time as

MMR vaccine, then varicella vaccine should be given at least 4 weeks later to avoid a weakening of the immune response to varicella vaccine caused by the MMR vaccine.

Adolescents (aged 13 to 19) and adults should receive 2 doses of vaccine, given 4 to 8 weeks apart.

Varicella vaccine is also recommended for **susceptible persons who have been exposed to chickenpox,** but only if they can be vaccinated within 72 hours after exposure. Vaccination within this time period will either prevent illness altogether, or significantly reduce the severity of illness.

The **duration of protection** is not yet known, but is at least 15 years. [See *The results of vaccination,* below, for more detail.]

Possible Side Effects of Varicella Vaccine

Giving varicella vaccine at the same time as other vaccines, such as MMR, does not increase the side effects of either vaccine.

Local/general reactions. Varicella vaccine is very safe. More than 15 million doses of the vaccine have been used in the United States since the vaccine was licensed there. Reactions are usually mild. Pain/soreness, redness, swelling, itching and/or rash at the site of injection occur in about 20% of children after a single dose of vaccine. The local reactions are almost always mild and brief in duration.

Fever less than 39°C (102°F) occurs in 15% of children following vaccination compared with 67% with chickenpox. A chickenpox-like rash, usually consisting of 10 pox or less, occurs in less than 5% of children after vaccination. There is no evidence that varicella vaccine causes serious adverse events.

Zoster after vaccination. Although rare, zoster (shingles) does occur after vaccination; the virus isolated from the skin rash has been shown to be the vaccine strain. However, follow-ups of 9,454 children participating in studies of varicella vaccine revealed that 8 cases of zoster occurred, a rate that is 4.3 times lower than the rate of zoster in children following natural chickenpox. Zoster in vaccinated children and adults has been mild and no chronic pain or other complications have been observed.

Transmission of the vaccine virus from healthy vaccinated children to susceptible contacts is a rare event. After more than 15 million doses of vaccine have been given in the United States, only 3 well-documented cases have been observed. Spread of the vaccine virus to susceptible persons occurs more commonly following vaccination of children with leukemia, but only if a rash develops after vaccination.

Reasons to Avoid or Delay Varicella Vaccine

Do not give. Varicella vaccine should not be given to
- *anyone with a history of allergy to any component of the vaccine,* including gelatin and neomycin. Having a history of contact dermatitis to neomycin is *not* a contraindication (i.e., the vaccine can be given to such a person).
- *immunocompromised persons.* Varicella vaccine is not licensed or recommended for persons with illnesses resulting in suppression of the immune system. However, its use in such persons may be beneficial; therefore, consultation with experts in immunosuppressive disorders and immunizations is advised. A research study is in progress involving persons with acute lymphoblastic leukemia and chickenpox vaccine. Additional information is available from the manufacturer.
- *pregnant women.* The effects of varicella vaccine on the fetus are unknown; therefore, this vaccine should not be given to pregnant women.

Do not delay. Vaccination should not be deferred or delayed because of minor illnesses, such as the common cold, with or without fever. Such infections do not increase the risk of side effects and do not interfere with the immune response to vaccination.

Delay. Moderate to severe illness, with or without fever, is a reason to delay routine immunization. This precaution may be taken in order to avoid the possibility of adding any side effects of the vaccine on top of the effects of the illness itself. However, if chickenpox infections are occurring in the community, vaccination is recommended because the risk of this type of infection in an unimmunized child is much greater than the risk of any side effects.

If the MMR and varicella vaccines are not given at the same time, they should be given at least 4 weeks apart. If given closer together, the immune response to some of the vaccines may be reduced.

The Results of Vaccination

Varicella vaccine induces antibody in more than 97% of healthy children after 1 dose and in adolescents and adults after 2 doses given 4 to 8 weeks apart. After 7 to 10 years, antibodies are as high after vaccination as they are after natural chickenpox in most children, but some lose antibodies and may become susceptible to chickenpox. Most such reinfections occur silently, but they may lead to a second case of chickenpox.

The current vaccine is 85–90% effective in preventing chickenpox and 100% effective in preventing moderate or severe disease in children. Children who develop chickenpox in spite of having been vaccinated have a mild illness compared with that experienced by children who have not been vaccinated: they have an average of less than 30 pox (compared to more than 300 with natural chickenpox), a lower occurrence of fever, and a more rapid recovery.

Evidence that varicella vaccine works includes the following:

- Controlled studies have demonstrated that the vaccine reduces the likelihood of getting chickenpox following exposure to an infected family member by over 97%.
- The reported rate of chickenpox has declined by more than 50% in the United States since the vaccine was introduced there.
- Follow-up of children years after vaccination has shown that protection against chickenpox following exposure to a case lasts 15 or more years.

The duration of protection is not yet known, but is at least 15 years. Neither the rate nor the severity of chickenpox increases with time since vaccination. Studies in Japan, where the vaccine has been in use longer than anywhere else, suggest that protection lasts more than 20 years.

Research is underway to determine whether varicella vaccine given to elderly persons will boost immunity and prevent zoster (shingles) in this group.

Summary

- In healthy children, varicella vaccine is very safe and very effective.
- Chickenpox can be a mild illness, but it can also result in severe damage and even death.
- Children who develop illness in spite of vaccination have very mild symptoms.
- Varicella vaccine is also effective in teenagers and adults who have not yet had chickenpox.
- Protection lasts at least 15 years, most likely at least 20 years, and possibly for life.
- The reactivated virus, zoster, is a problem particularly for older persons, who are most likely to suffer complications and least likely to recover from infection.

- Chickenpox is a costly disease. Parents of infected children incur the largest proportion of costs.
- Studies are in progress in a number of areas to determine the extent of effectiveness in preventing illness in groups at risk (e.g., elderly persons, persons with suppressed immunity).

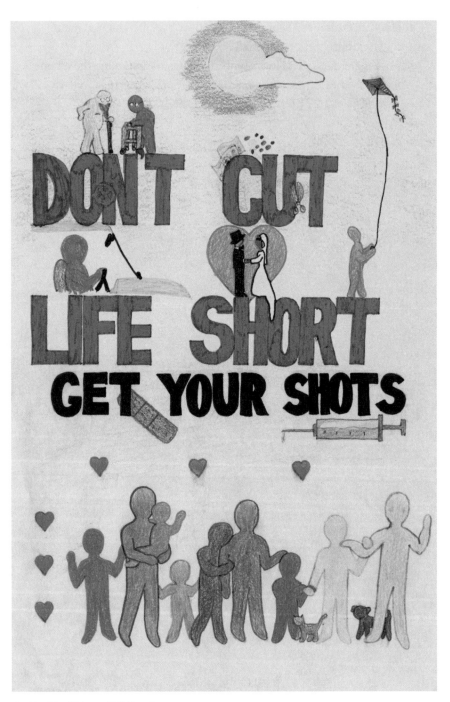

Sue Hee Kim, Richmond Hill, Ontario

CHAPTER 16

Vaccines for Foreign Travel and for the Future

The previous chapters have covered the routine vaccines recommended for all children. This chapter offers an overview of some of the other vaccines currently available as well as vaccines that are at various stages of development.

Vaccines for Foreign Travel

The four vaccines discussed in this chapter are recommended for travellers who will be visiting parts of the world where certain infections are much more common than they are in Canada.

The following vaccines are not recommended for routine use in children or adults in Canada because the frequency of infection with these diseases is quite low in this country:
- hepatitis A vaccine;
- typhoid vaccine;
- yellow fever vaccine;
- Japanese encephalitis vaccine.

Each of the three sections below lists groups that should receive the vaccine. For specific advice about which vaccines may be necessary in certain countries and whether they are suitable for children, contact your physician or the local medical officer of health.

Hepatitis A Vaccine

The virus. Hepatitis A is one of several viruses that infects the liver. The liver is the major chemical factory of the body:
- It completes the digestion of food begun in the stomach and intestines, changing the food into forms that can be used by various tissues.
- It stores sugar, fat and certain vitamins.
- It breaks down many chemicals and toxins so that they can be excreted by the body.

Healthy carriers. Many people do not know they have been infected with hepatitis A because they do not get sick. Such people are known as healthy carriers. Infection *without* illness is quite common in infants and young children. Although not visibly sick, the children are infectious and spread the virus to others. The virus is excreted in feces and can be spread by contaminated hands, food and water.

The illness. Adults are much more likely to become ill when infected. Symptoms include fever, fatigue, loss of appetite, nausea, vomiting, abdominal pain, and yellow skin and eyes (jaundice). The illness may last several weeks, but most people recover completely. No treatment is available for this infection.

On occasion, the infection causes such severe liver damage that the person dies. Unlike hepatitis B, hepatitis A virus does not cause chronic infection of the liver, cirrhosis (scarring of the liver) or liver cancer. Immunity after infection lasts for life.

The vaccine. Hepatitis A vaccine is a **killed intact virus vaccine**. The virus is grown in tissue culture cells, purified and then killed with formalin (formaldehyde). Several different vaccines are available. The manufacturing processes differ slightly, as do the administration schedules (i.e., either 1 or 2 doses are required).

Results. The vaccines have been more than 90% effective in preventing infection with hepatitis A. Immunity is expected to last many years after vaccination. It is not yet known whether boosters will be required. Other than mild pain and redness at the injection site, side effects are uncommon.

Recommendations. Hepatitis A vaccine is recommended for persons travelling to parts of the world where hepatitis is a common infection (e.g., Latin America, Africa, Asia). It is also recommended:
- for children and adults living in areas in Canada where the infection is common (e.g., areas with poor sanitation and unsafe water supplies);
- for certain groups at high risk of infection (e.g., drug users, men who have sex with men);
- for persons infected with hepatitis C virus, because the risk of *severe* hepatitis A infection is high in this group;
- for control of outbreaks of hepatitis A infection in childcare centres and other institutions where people (particularly children) are in frequent close contact in a confined setting (e.g., prisons, orphanages, schools, camps).

For outbreaks in childcare settings, the children, parents, siblings and staff should be vaccinated. Usually when young children get infected, they don't get sick, but they spread the virus to adults who do get sick when infected.

Because of insufficient information on the use of the vaccine in children less than 1 year of age, the vaccine is not recommended for very young children.

Typhoid Vaccine

Typhoid fever is now rare in Canada and other developed countries. Most cases involve persons who have travelled to underdeveloped parts of the world where sanitation is poor, and food and water are often contaminated.

The bacteria. Typhoid fever is a severe infection caused by a bacterium called *Salmonella typhi*. The infection can be acquired by close contact with an infected person (e.g., spread from person to person if hands are not washed properly after bowel movements), or by eating food or drinking water contaminated with the bacteria. Bacteria spreading from the intestines into the bloodstream causes infection.

The illness. Symptoms of the disease include high fever for a week or more, cough and abdominal pain. Treatment with antibiotics is very effective, although many strains, especially in developing countries, have become resistant to commonly used antibiotics.

The vaccine. Two different typhoid vaccines are available in Canada: live attenuated (weakened) oral vaccine and purified polysaccharide vaccine. They are equally effective. Here's the difference between the two: the first one contains live, weakened bacteria and is taken orally (by mouth) in the form of large capsules; several doses are required. The purified polysaccharide vaccine doesn't contain live bacteria and is given as an injection; only one shot is required.

Live, attenuated oral vaccine. Unlike most vaccines, this one is taken orally. It consists of a genetically changed strain of typhoid bacteria. The vaccine strain, in its attenuated (weakened) state, multiplies briefly in the intestinal tract, then dies. Because the vaccine strain dies before being excreted, the vaccine strain cannot spread to others. The vaccine bacteria do not invade the body and do not cause typhoid fever. The vaccine is produced in the form of capsules, which are swallowed. One capsule is taken every other day, for a total of four capsules. They must be stored in the refrigerator, otherwise the live bacteria in the vaccine may die and the vaccine will not work.

Results. The vaccine is 40–65% effective in preventing typhoid fever. Some people experience side effects such as mild nausea and abdominal distress. A booster is recommended after 7 years if exposure to typhoid continues.

Recommendations. The capsules containing the vaccine are quite large and therefore difficult for some people to swallow. For this reason, the vaccine is recommended only for adults and children over 6 years old who can swallow the capsules. [See Text Box below for general recommendation.]

Purified polysaccharide vaccine. This vaccine is made of a sugar (polysaccharide) that forms the outer coat of the typhoid bacteria. The polysaccharide is extracted from the bacteria and purified to make the vaccine. There is no risk of infection from the vaccine because it doesn't contain live bacteria. A single dose of vaccine is given by injection.

General recommendation

The typhoid vaccine is recommended only for travellers who will be at high risk of exposure (e.g., those who will be living/working in rural areas with poor sanitation) in countries with a high rate of typhoid fever. Tourists visiting resort hotels for short periods in such countries are *not* at high risk.

Results. The vaccine is at least 55–75% effective. Boosters are recommended after 3 years if exposure to typhoid continues.

Recommendations. This vaccine is not recommended for children under 2 years of age because of insufficient information on safety and effectiveness for that age group. [See the Text Box above for general recommendation.]

Yellow Fever and Japanese Encephalitis Vaccines

The viruses. Both yellow fever and Japanese encephalitis are infections caused by viruses that are found only in certain parts of the world. The two viruses are spread by mosquitoes.

The illnesses. Infection with *yellow fever virus* can cause
* hepatitis (acute inflammation of the liver). The symptoms are similar to those of hepatitis from many other sources (e.g., hepatitis A, B, C, D). Symptoms are caused by malfunction of the liver;
* bleeding (from the nose, mouth, intestinal tract and skin, and even into the lungs);
* death (the death rate is as high as 20%).

Infection with *Japanese encephalitis virus* can cause encephalitis, which means inflammation of the brain. Encephalitis occurs in only a small proportion of infected persons though. Most people get a flu-like illness with fever, aches and pains. Symptoms of encephalitis include fever, severe headache, vomiting, convulsions and decreased level of consciousness.

Many different viruses can cause encephalitis. Japanese encephalitis refers to encephalitis caused by the Japanese encephalitis virus. The viruses causing encephalitis are all different from each other; many were named after the place where they were first isolated, such as Japan, California, LaCrosse, Murray Valley and West Nile.

The vaccines. *Yellow fever vaccine* is a live attenuated (weakened) virus vaccine. *Japanese encephalitis vaccine* is a purified, inactivated vaccine prepared from brain tissue of mice infected with Japanese encephalitis virus.

Results. Both vaccines are very effective in preventing disease.

Recommendations. These vaccines are recommended only for those who will be at risk of infection because of travel to parts of the world where these viruses exist. Neither vaccine is recommended for infants less than 6 months of age because of uncertainty as to safety and effectiveness at that age.

Vaccines for the Future

The vaccines described briefly below are being developed for the future.

RSV Vaccine

- Respiratory syncytial virus (RSV) is an extremely common infection. Almost all children are infected by 2 years of age. Outbreaks occur every winter.
- It causes serious lung infections in the first year of life as well as in the elderly. RSV can cause a severe, even fatal, illness if it occurs in a young infant (less than 6 months of age).
- The hospitalization and mortality rates from RSV in the elderly (persons aged 65 and over) are almost as great as those for influenza.
- Complications are similar to those of influenza.
- Infection with RSV does not produce long-lasting immunity.
- People become infected with RSV almost every time they are exposed to it. Repeat infections are usually much less severe than the first infection.
- The vaccine is in the early stages of research at this time.

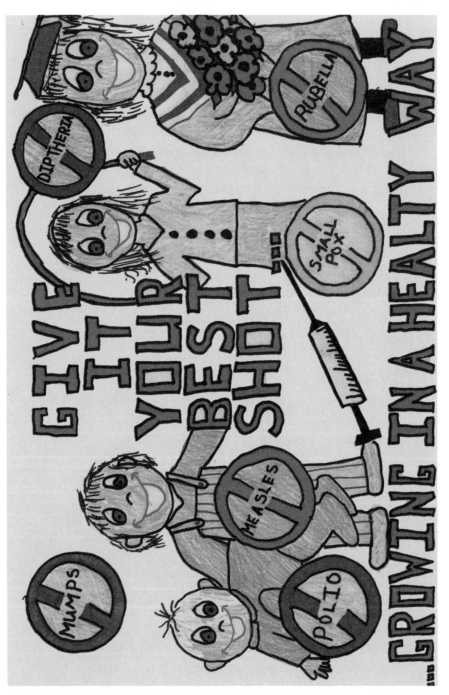

Trina Lewis, Dowling, Ontario

Rotavirus Vaccine

- Rotavirus is the most common cause of acute diarrhea in infants and young children.
- It causes severe, watery diarrhea and high fever. If fluid intake is not maintained, dehydration can develop rapidly, leading to death.
- In less developed countries, rotavirus diarrhea is a major cause of death.
- Immunity after infection does not last long, but repeat infections are usually less severe than the first infection.
- A live, attenuated (weakened) rotavaccine was licensed in the United States in 1999. It was discontinued because of concern that it might cause intussusception (a form of bowel obstruction).
- Research continues with more weakened versions of the vaccine so that they can be used safely in less developed countries.

HIV Vaccine

- Development of a vaccine to prevent or treat human immuno-deficiency virus (HIV) infection and AIDS has been slow. The virus that causes HIV changes so rapidly that it escapes control by the immune system.

Hepatitis C Vaccine

- Hepatitis C is a virus that causes chronic infection of the liver. This leads to liver damage and liver cancer.
- Until the hepatitis C virus can be grown in the laboratory, the vaccine cannot be developed.

Group A Streptococcal Vaccine

- Group A streptococcus causes strep throat, impetigo, acute rheumatic fever and acute nephritis (inflammation of the kidneys).
- Complications of group A strep infection, such as rheumatic fever, are now rare in North America and Western Europe. However, they are still common in many parts of the world.

- Acute rheumatic fever can lead to permanent damage of heart valves and chronic heart disease.
- A vaccine that would prevent such complications will be very useful.

Group B Streptococcal Vaccine

- Group B streptococcus is a very common cause of severe infections among newborn infants, especially premature infants.
- This bacteria causes bacteremia, pneumonia, and meningitis in newborns and young infants.

CHAPTER 17

Questions and Answers About Vaccination

1 What should I do if my child has a reaction to vaccination?

General

After immunization, children may cry and be fussy because of pain at the injection site (i.e., where they got the shot). A few children also develop fever, but high fever (greater than 40°C or 104°F) is unusual with any of the current vaccines. Read on to find out what you can do to relieve mild reactions such as pain, fussiness and low fever.

If your child seems really sick or if you are worried *at all* about how your child looks or feels, call your child's doctor!

Crying, fussiness

If your child is crying a lot or is very fussy, you can give him or her a medicine called acetaminophen, which helps to reduce pain and fever. Some brand names of acetaminophen are Tylenol, Panadol and Tempra. [See Table 17.1 below, for the proper dose of acetaminophen for your child.]

Do not give aspirin (acetylsalicylic acid, ASA) for pain or fever because its use in children has been associated with an increased risk of Reye's syndrome, a severe disorder of the liver and brain.

 Call your child's doctor if the crying or fussiness lasts more than 24 hours.

TABLE 17.1

Dose of acetaminophen* for infants and children, by age and weight

DOSE OF ACETAMINOPHEN THAT CAN BE GIVEN EVERY 4 TO 6 HOURS				
1–3 months	**4–11 months**	**12–23 months**	**2–3 years**	**4–5 years**
2.7–5.4 kg	5.5–8.1 kg	8.2–10.9 kg	11.0–16.3 kg	16.4–21.8 kg
(6–11 lbs.)	*(12–17 lbs.)*	*(18–23 lbs.)*	*(24–35 lbs.)*	*(36–47 lbs.)*
½ dropperful infant drops	1 dropperful infant drops or ½ teaspoon children's liquid	1-½ dropperfuls infant drops or ¼ teaspoon children's liquid	2 chewable 80 mg tablets or 1 teaspoon children's liquid	3 chewable 80 mg tablets or 1-½ teaspoons children's liquid

* *The dose of acetaminophen is 15 mg per kilogram of weight. Approximate doses are given in the Table, based on age and weight.*
Infant drops contain 80 mg of acetaminophen per ml.
Children's liquid contains 160 mg of acetaminophen per 5 ml (5 ml=1 teaspoon).
Chewable tablets contain either 80 mg or 160 mg of acetaminophen.

Fever

If you think your child has a fever, check your child's temperature — don't guess. The most accurate way to do this in a young child is by taking a rectal temperature. (Be sure to use a lubricant, such as petroleum jelly, when doing so.) Digital thermometers are preferred to glass mercury thermometers for safety reasons.

To reduce fever:
- Give your child plenty to drink.
- Clothe your child lightly. Do not cover or wrap your child tightly!
- Give your child acetaminophen. [See Table 17.1 for guidelines on doses.]

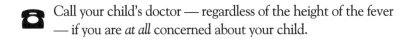 Call your child's doctor — regardless of the height of the fever — if you are *at all* concerned about your child.

Swelling

If your child's injection site (leg or arm) is swollen, hot, red and/or tender to touch, try these tips to relieve the discomfort:
- Apply a clean, cool washcloth for 15 to 20 minutes over the sore area.
- Give acetaminophen.

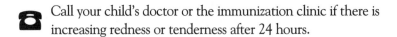 Call your child's doctor or the immunization clinic if there is increasing redness or tenderness after 24 hours.

2 How serious are the infections discussed in this book?

Each vaccine has been developed to prevent a certain disease (e.g., measles, diphtheria, chickenpox). All of the target diseases can be very serious and most can lead to death — even with today's advanced medical care. [See Table 17.2, under Question 8, for a summary of diseases and vaccines.]

Diphtheria

Diphtheria still kills about 1 out of 10 people who get it. It can damage the heart muscle and lead to death. Diphtheria bacteria still occur in Canada. There is a direct relationship between the rates of immunization and disease: whenever the rate of immunization against diphtheria declines, the rates of diphtheria cases and deaths increase.

Tetanus

Tetanus spores are in dust and soil everywhere. If these spores get into a wound (no matter how small), tetanus bacteria may grow and release toxin (poison) in the body. Tetanus is a very serious disease. Even with modern treatment, tetanus still kills 10–20% of those infected.

Pertussis

Pertussis remains a serious illness in infants. Babies with pertussis cough for 6 weeks or more and often lose weight because of feeding problems and vomiting. They also have a high rate of ear and lung infections. In Canada, about 20–30% of infants with pertussis (or about 1 in 4) are admitted to hospital. Of these infants, 1 in 400 dies and about 1 in 400 suffers permanent brain damage.

Children who have pertussis in infancy are more likely to have learning and behaviour problems than children who did not get the disease. Pertussis also occurs in older children, adolescents and adults. Although complications are much less frequent in such persons than in infants, the illness can cause several weeks of severe spells of coughing and result in absences from school or work. Adolescents and adults with pertussis are a very common source of infection for infants.

Polio

Polio can cause paralysis of various parts of the body, including nerve centres controlling breathing, circulation and other vital functions. Death can occur. Paralytic polio has been eradicated from the Western Hemisphere, Western Europe and East Asia by vaccination of children; but it still occurs in other parts of the world. We must continue to vaccinate children because of the risk of travellers bringing poliovirus back to Canada.

Haemophilus influenzae type b (Hib)

Before routine vaccination, about 1 in every 300 Canadian children developed meningitis or other severe Hib infections by 5 years of age. Even with treatment, Hib meningitis killed 1 in 20 children and caused detectable brain damage in 1 in 3 survivors. Hib can also cause serious infections of the throat, lungs, blood, joints and bones.

Measles

Many of those opposed to vaccination claim that measles is not as serious as stated by public health authorities. They say, "Everyone I know survived measles in their childhood." For a lot of people, this statement is true; but many children did not survive the disease. No one claims that there is a high death rate from measles in Canada. But measles is a serious illness, even in healthy, well-nourished children.

Complications such as ear infections and bacterial pneumonia occur in 1 out of 10 children. Encephalitis occurs in about 1 out of 1,000 cases; it causes death in one-third of these cases and severe brain damage in another third. Measles causes subacute sclerosing panencephalitis (SSPE) in about 1 in 100,000 cases. SSPE occurs years after the attack of measles and leads to seizures, dementia, coma and death (always) because of progressive destruction of brain cells.

Mumps

Mumps is usually not a severe illness in children, but can cause deafness, meningitis and encephalitis. It can also cause inflammation of the testicles (orchitis) in older boys and adult men, which can lead to sterility.

Rubella

The most serious complication of rubella occurs if a woman becomes infected during pregnancy. If a woman gets rubella during the first 20 weeks of pregnancy, the risk of death or severe malformations of her baby is very high.

Hepatitis B

Hepatitis B is usually not a severe illness in children. However, 9 out of every 10 children who are infected at birth will develop chronic infection of the liver. These chronic infections often lead to scarring of the liver and liver cancer later in life. Both of these liver diseases are usually fatal.

Influenza

Influenza is usually not a severe illness in children. But severe complications may occur in healthy infants and in children of any age with chronic heart and lung disorders. School-age children are the major source of spread of influenza in the community.

Chickenpox

Chickenpox is considered by most to be a mild childhood disease. However, the disease bears significant costs — both health-related and financial. Complications can result from chickenpox (pneumonia, encephalitis and cerebellar ataxia), some of which can lead to death. There is also a high price tag associated with the illness itself, even for uncomplicated cases: costs of visits to doctors and medications; days lost from childcare or school; and the time and salary lost by parents who stay home to care for the sick child.

The disease is much more severe in adolescents and adults, so these age groups have higher rates of complications and death from chickenpox than do younger age groups.

Pneumococcal infections

The pneumococcus bacterium is the most common cause of serious bacterial infections in children. It causes meningitis, pneumonia and bacteremia. Each of these serious infections can kill or cause permanent damage if not diagnosed and treated promptly.

Meningococcal infections

The meningococcus bacterium causes meningitis and septicemia. It kills about 10% of people who get the infection, even with prompt diagnosis and treatment. Outbreaks can occur in schools and universities/colleges.

3 Weren't some of these diseases disappearing long before vaccines became available?

No. A common argument of those opposed to immunization is that these infections were declining in frequency in Canada and other developed countries long before vaccines became available. This is not true. Until vaccines became available, there was no significant change in the *number of cases* of diphtheria, tetanus, pertussis, polio, measles, mumps, rubella, Hib or hepatitis B.

What was changing before vaccines became available was the *death rate* from some of these infections. Improvements in social and economic conditions led to declining death rates for many common infections. Children who are healthy and well-nourished are much less likely than malnourished children to die from measles or pertussis.

In short, these improvements did not prevent all disease or deaths. Before vaccines, the frequency of the infections remained the same, but the risk of death from infection decreased. [See Table 17.2, under Question 8, for a summary of diseases and vaccines.]

4 Won't breastfeeding and good nutrition prevent these childhood infections?

Breastfeeding is not an alternative to infant vaccination, and it does not enhance the responses to vaccination. Breastfeeding provides some protection against many infections because special antibodies are made in the breast and are present in human breast milk. Babies who are breastfed generally have lower rates of many infections, including viral respiratory infections, ear infections and diarrhea. The protection provided by breast milk is incomplete and can be overcome if the baby is exposed to a large amount of a germ. Moreover, the protection disappears rapidly as soon as breastfeeding stops.

Good nutrition helps the body's defences against infection to function normally. Infections are more severe in anyone with poor nutrition. Special immune cells called lymphocytes are easily damaged if one's diet does not include enough protein. For this reason, malnourished children are much more likely to die of infections such as measles or pertussis than well-nourished children. Vitamin A deficiency, in particular, greatly increases the risk of severe illness.

5 Aren't the only children who die of these infections suffering from malnutrition or defects of the immune system?

Although infections such as measles and pertussis are much more likely to kill a child who is malnourished or who has immune system defects, these infections can also kill healthy, well-nourished children. Malnutrition was not a contributing factor in the deaths of any of the children who died of pertussis in the United States in the 1990s.

6 Do vaccines really work?

Yes!

All vaccine-preventable diseases have declined significantly in countries with successful immunization programs. Wherever vaccination rates are high, disease rates are low. Conversely, when vaccination rates decline (often because of fear of unproven dangers of vaccines), the diseases and related deaths increase in frequency.

Smallpox was the first disease to disappear because of vaccination. There have been no cases of smallpox anywhere in the world since 1979!

Paralytic polio has been eliminated from most of the world by vaccination. A global vaccination program is expected to completely eradicate the disease within the next 5 to 10 years. [See Table 17.2, under Question 8, for a summary of diseases and vaccines.]

7 Is there a risk of catching the illness from the vaccine itself?

Inactivated vaccines (such as inactivated polio and influenza vaccines) and **purified vaccines** (such as diphtheria and tetanus toxoids, and Hib, acellular pertussis, pneumococcal, meningococcal and hepatitis B vaccines) *do not* have any living germs in them. These vaccines stimulate the immune system, but they cannot cause the infection.

Live, attenuated vaccines (such as measles, mumps and rubella vaccines) *do* infect cells and multiply in the body. The vaccine viruses have been sufficiently weakened (attenuated) in the laboratory that they stimulate immunity without causing a full-blown infection. Measles, mumps and rubella vaccine viruses do not spread from a vaccinated child to another person. Chickenpox vaccine is also a live, attenuated vaccine. Spread of this vaccine virus may occur after vaccination of healthy children, but such spread is extremely rare. However, the vaccine virus can sometimes spread from a vaccinated child who has leukemia to other children.

Oral polio vaccine (OPV), however, not only infects the intestinal tract, but is also excreted in the feces. The vaccine strains can spread from person to person (for example, by touching a feces-contaminated surface or object). Such spread is usually helpful, though, because those who get the polio vaccine virus this way may also become immunized.

OPV is a very safe and effective vaccine. There is, however, an incredibly small risk of getting paralytic polio from the vaccine. The most recent estimate of the risk of vaccine-associated paralytic polio after the first dose of OPV (given to infants) is 1 out of every 1.3 million doses. The risk is much smaller for susceptible persons exposed to a vaccinated child.

To avoid the very small risk of disease associated with the oral vaccine, Canadian provinces and territories that did use the live OPV switched to the **inactivated polio vaccine (IPV)** during the 1990s. Since 1997, only IPV has been used in Canada. Experts are confident that the switch to IPV will maintain the remarkable accomplishment of eradication of paralytic polio in the Western Hemisphere. [See Table 17.2, under Question 8, for a summary of diseases and vaccines.]

8 What about the risk of side effects from vaccines?

The risks associated with vaccines are much, much less than the risks associated with the diseases themselves. [See Table 17.2 below for a summary of diseases and vaccines.] The following facts highlight the risks of both the diseases and the vaccines.

Fever

Fever can occur after vaccination and may cause convulsions (seizures) in a few cases. Febrile seizures (those caused by high fever) do not cause permanent brain damage, retardation, learning problems or behaviour problems, and they do not increase the risk of epilepsy or any other brain disorder. The risk of convulsions is much higher after natural measles or pertussis disease than after vaccination.

Pertussis

Pertussis kills 1 to 3 infants every year in Canada and an equal number suffer severe brain damage. Brain damage after pertussis vaccine is extremely rare, if it occurs at all.

Measles

Measles causes encephalitis (inflammation of the brain) in about 1 out of 1,000 cases. One-third of those with measles encephalitis die and one-third survive with brain damage. Encephalitis occurs about once in every 1 million measles vaccinations. This occurrence rate is so low that it is unclear whether the vaccine or some other infection is responsible.

Mumps

Meningitis occurs in 1 in 10 cases of mumps. Meningitis occurs after 1 in 800,000 mumps vaccinations.

Rubella

If a woman becomes infected during the first 20 weeks of pregnancy, chances are high (8 out of 10) that the fetus will also be infected. Joint pain affects twice as many women with natural infection as women who are vaccinated.

Diphtheria and tetanus

Diphtheria kills 1 in every 10 persons who get the illness; tetanus kills up to 1 in 5. Serious reactions after either vaccine are extremely rare.

Hib disease, and meningococcal and pneumococcal diseases

The bacteria at the source of these illnesses cause bacterial meningitis and other life-threatening infections, such as bacteremia (infection of the blood) and pneumonia. Even with treatment, 5–20% of children with bacterial meningitis die and a similar proportion of survivors sustain deafness and other forms of brain damage. The vaccines are extremely safe; serious reactions are very rare, if they occur at all.

TABLE 17.2

Summary of diseases and vaccines, Canada

DISEASE	AVERAGE NUMBER OF CASES AND RELATED DEATHS (per year)		EFFECTS OF DISEASE	SIDE EFFECTS OF VACCINE
	Before vaccine	After vaccine		
Diphtheria	12,000 cases with 1,000 deaths	0–5 cases with 0 deaths	Severe sore throat, marked weakness, nerve damage, heart failure. Death in 10%.	DTaP vaccine: 20% of infants have local redness, pain; less than 5% have fever; more redness and swelling with booster at 4–6 years.
Tetanus	60–75 cases with 40–50 deaths	0–2 cases and no deaths since 1991	Toxin affects spinal cord leading to painful muscle spasms and seizures.	See above for DTaP. Local redness and pain common with adult booster.
Pertussis	30,000–50,000 cases with 50–100 deaths	3,000 cases with 1–5 deaths	Severe spasms of cough lasting 3–6 weeks, pneumonia, convulsions. Brain damage or death in 1 of every 400 infants.	See above for DTaP. The risk of brain damage after pertussis vaccine is too small to be measured.
Polio	2,000 cases in last epidemic in 1959	0	Muscle paralysis in 1 out of 100 persons infected with polio. Death in severe cases.	Inactivated polio vaccine (IPV) is used in Canada. No risk of disease from vaccine. Given combined with DTaP (see above for side effects).
Hib	1,500 cases of meningitis and 1,500 cases of infections of blood, bone, lung, skin, joints	About 30 cases	Meningitis kills in 5% of cases and leads to brain damage and deafness in 10–15% of survivors.	Given in combination with DTaP/IPV (see above for side effects).
Measles	95% of children have measles by age 18, or 300,000 cases with 300 deaths and 300 children with brain damage	Less than 50 cases with 0 deaths	Severe bronchitis, high fever, rash for 7–14 days; death in 1 per 1,000 cases; encephalitis in 1 per 1,000 cases.	Given combined with mumps and rubella vaccines (MMR). 5–10% have fever with or without rash 8–10 days after vaccine. No risk of disease from vaccine. Risk of encephalitis 1 case per 1 million doses. 1 in 24,000 develops low platelets.
Mumps	30,000 cases	95 cases	Fever, swollen salivary glands. No visible illness in more than 50% of cases. Encephalitis in 1 per 200 cases; deafness in 1 per 200,000 cases.	See MMR above.
Rubella	85% of children have rubella by age 20, or 250,000 cases. About 200 cases of congenital rubella syndrome.	25 cases. 0–3 babies with congenital rubella syndrome born to unvaccinated mothers.	Fever, swollen glands, rash. No symptoms in about 50% of cases. Severe damage to fetus if mother infected during first trimester of pregnancy.	See MMR above. Congenital rubella syndrome has not been observed after vaccination of pregnant women. 25% of vaccinated adult women have joint pain.

9 Why do some children who have been vaccinated still get measles?

Opponents of vaccination are quick to point out that many cases of measles occur in vaccinated children. They claim this proves that the vaccine doesn't work. In outbreaks of measles in Canada and the United States in the 1990s, it is true that more than half of the cases occurred in school-age children who had been given measles vaccine. But to say that this means that the vaccine doesn't work is incorrect. This argument is too simplistic, and it uses faulty logic.

We know that 1 dose of measles vaccine is not 100% effective. We know that about 5–10% of children are not protected after a single dose of vaccine. Let's use these facts in an example.

Example

In a school with 1,000 students, assume 95% of children get vaccinated. This means that there are 950 vaccinated children and 50 unvaccinated children. The number of children who are still susceptible to measles is 145 — 50 unvaccinated children plus 10% of the 950 vaccinated children who are unprotected after 1 dose (or 95).

One child in the school comes back from a holiday with measles. Measles is so contagious that it quickly spreads in the school. One-half of the 145 susceptible children catch it: half of the 50 unvaccinated children (or 25) get measles and half of the 95 vaccine-failure children (or 47) get measles. Therefore, there are 72 cases of measles. The proportion of cases that occurred in vaccinated children is 47 of the total 72, or 65%! This seems very high, but it does not mean that the vaccine works only 65% of the time.

Whenever a vaccine is not 100% effective and most children have been vaccinated, more cases will occur in vaccinated than in unvaccinated children during outbreaks, only because there *are* more vaccinated than unvaccinated children.

The 25 cases of measles in the unvaccinated group came from a total of 50 children; the attack rate in this group is 50%. The 47 cases among vaccine failures came from a total of 950 children, an attack rate of only 4.9%.

From these numbers, we can see that unvaccinated children were 10 times more likely to catch measles! The vaccine was 90% effective. This is the commonly observed figure when only 1 dose of measles vaccine is given. When 2 doses are routinely given to children, the vaccine is nearly 100% effective and outbreaks no longer occur among vaccinated children.

10 If the first dose of measles vaccine doesn't work, won't a second dose also fail?

The main reason infants fail to respond to measles vaccine is the presence of antibody to measles, which infants get from their mothers during pregnancy. It takes only a very small amount of antibody to kill the measles vaccine virus. (If the immune system kills the vaccine virus, the vaccine will not induce immunity to natural measles virus.) About 5% of infants still have enough measles antibody at 12 months of age to do just that.

Studies of children who failed to respond to the first dose of vaccine at 12 to 15 months of age have shown that over 99% of them *did* respond normally to the second dose. Studies of outbreaks in schools have confirmed that measles is very rare in children who have had 2 doses of measles vaccine.

11 Why do chiropractors and homeopaths advise against vaccination?

Although some chiropractors and homeopathic physicians are against vaccination, the policy of the Faculty of Homeopathy at the Royal

London Homeopathic Hospital is as follows: "Where there is no medical contraindication, immunization should be carried out in the normal way using conventional tested and approved vaccines." The Canadian College of Chiropractic also recommends that all children should receive routine immunization.

Different views of "natural" and "beneficial"

Many believers in homeopathy, naturopathy and other alternative systems of medicine seem to believe that nature's way is best and that "foreign," "unnatural" or "artificial" things like vaccines should be avoided. It is difficult to comprehend why a disease like measles is considered "natural" and "beneficial" when it kills and damages so many children — even healthy, well-nourished children.

The only infections that are natural and beneficial are those that lead to the successful growth and multiplication of many kinds of bacteria within our bodies within a few days of birth. These bacteria are called "normal flora" because they live on our skin and within us on the lining of the nose, throat, stomach and intestines without making us sick. They are beneficial to us because they make it harder for harmful bacteria to infect us. They are also beneficial because they help make certain vitamins for us from chemicals in our food.

The bacteria and viruses that make us sick are part of nature, but like many things in nature, they are harmful, not helpful. Being natural is not always good for human beings.

Vaccines are also part of nature. Some vaccines are made from live viruses that have undergone natural mutations (weakenings). They have been altered so that they no longer make us sick but still induce immunity to the natural, "wild" virus. Other vaccines are actually chemicals that have been extracted or purified from viruses or bacteria. When injected into the body, they stimulate the immune system in a way very similar to the infection, again without making us sick.

12 How can immunity that results from immunization be as good as immunity from natural infection?

Opponents of vaccination often claim that natural immunity (from an infection) is better than immunity from a vaccine. Immunity after most vaccines is just as effective as that induced by disease. As well, every infection described in this book has a great risk of causing harm. The truth is that the proven risk of damage and death caused by the disease is *far* worse than the so-called "benefit" of obtaining immunity through disease.

To understand that the two ways of achieving immunity are equally effective, you must first understand how the immune system works. An overview is presented below.

How the immune system works

There are two functions of the immune system: immediate response and long-term response. The immediate response kills infectious germs and promotes recovery from the infection. The long-term response maintains immunity so that the person will be protected against infection if exposed to the germs in the future.

Immediate response

The parts of the immune system involved in destroying bad germs are called antibodies and lymphocytes. Antibodies are proteins made by immune cells. The antibodies attach to the surface of the germ and kill it, either by damaging it directly or by allowing other white blood cells to kill the germ. Lymphocytes (white blood cells) can attack some germs directly. Usually, though, lymphocytes work indirectly by killing the cells that are infected with the germ.

It takes time for the body to develop an immediate immune response. So, with natural infection, sometimes the infection kills the person or causes severe damage before the immune response kicks in.

Vaccines are used to stimulate both antibodies and lymphocytes so that they are present in the body *before* exposure to an infection occurs. Following vaccination, the immune system responds as if infection has occurred. There may be a difference in the *amount* of antibody made after infection compared with after vaccine, but the same *kinds* of antibodies and immune cells are made. The antibodies and lymphocytes produced in both cases target the identical chemicals on the surface of the germ.

Long-term response

The second function of the immune system is to establish immune memory. When we say a person is immune to a certain disease, we mean that immune memory against that particular infection has been established. Special lymphocytes, called memory cells, are stimulated by both infection and vaccination. These memory cells live (remain active) for a very long time, perhaps even for life. If a person with established immunity to a certain infection is exposed to that infection again, the active memory cells respond very quickly and signal both the cells that make antibodies and the cells that attack germs to get to work.

It is important to note, however, that each type of infectious germ is attacked by a separate, distinct set of antibodies and lymphocytes. Immunity to one infection does not "create" immunity to other infections. Antibodies and lymphocytes made in response to measles infection or measles vaccine react only to measles virus. Memory cells for rubella infection will not activate antibody to fight against diphtheria.

In summary, immunity induced by vaccines is as effective as immunity induced by disease, without the risk of disease.

13   Does immunity wear off over time?

The levels of antibody in the blood decline over time following both natural infection and vaccination. But even though antibodies disappear, immune memory persists. Most vaccines produce immune memory that lasts a very long time, if not for life.

But others, for example diphtheria and tetanus toxoids, must be repeated every 10 years to maintain protection against diphtheria and tetanus. These repeated shots are called boosters. When a booster is given to a person who already has immune memory (perhaps from a previous booster), the immune response creates antibody (necessary to fight infection) much faster and stronger than when a booster is given to a person with no immune memory.

In other words, the process of building immunity takes longer in a person who has never been exposed to the infection before. In the time it takes this person's immune system to build immunity against a particular germ, that germ can do lots of damage.

14   Won't adults be at risk of catching these infections if immunity wears off?

Infections such as measles, mumps, rubella and chickenpox are more severe in adults than in children. Therefore, there is some concern that adults might be at risk if immunity from childhood vaccination wears off. Natural infections with measles, mumps and rubella do induce lifelong immunity.

Vaccination also produces very long-lasting immunity. Immune memory resulting from vaccination seems to persist even if there is no antibody detectable in the blood. The occurrence rate of measles, mumps, rubella and chickenpox among those who were the first to be vaccinated has not been affected by the passage of time.

The medical surveillance system in Canada maintains a watch on the occurrence of many infectious diseases [see Chapter 2]. This complex reporting network detects changes in the frequency of infections occurring in the North American population. If infections are beginning to occur in adults who were vaccinated as children, the network will respond by adjusting the vaccination program appropriately (e.g., adding booster doses of a vaccine).

Some boosters are necessary

Although diphtheria and tetanus are also severe diseases in adults, they are somewhat different from most other infections in the way they cause disease. Both of these diseases cause illness by producing a toxin (or poison). Protection against these diseases requires the actual presence of antibody in the blood at the time a person is exposed to the toxin.

Even though immune memory lasts 40 years or more after vaccination, antibody levels decrease over time. These infectious toxins are so potent that disease can occur before the immune system has time to respond. Adults must receive boosters every 10 years to be protected against diphtheria and tetanus. They shouldn't wait until there is a need.

Keep vaccinations up-to-date

After vaccination, patients are given a card to record the date and vaccine received. These cards are a record of vaccination and should be kept up-to-date, in a safe place.

15 Can vaccines "wear out" the immune system?

The human immune system has a truly enormous capacity to recognize different proteins and other chemicals called antigens. It can respond to intense and repeated stimulation. The food we eat, the air we breathe and the water we drink every day is filled with antigens that our immune system recognizes as foreign. Its job is to make appropriate responses to help the body get rid of any foreign substances.

High tolerance levels

The challenge that vaccination presents to the immune system is not likely to be a significant addition to the daily load of foreign antigens entering the body, even for a 2-month-old baby. Scientists have estimated that infants have the capacity to respond to about 10,000 different antigens at any one time.

The vaccines used today are much more highly purified than those used in the past, so even though infants and children now receive more vaccines than they did 30 years ago, the total amount of proteins and polysaccharides the immune system must deal with is still much lower than it used to be.

Study of frequent vaccination

A study of the effects of repeated immunization with several vaccines was carried out with a group of employees who worked at the United States Army Biological Warfare Research Laboratory in Maryland. The employees had frequently been vaccinated with many routine and experimental vaccines to protect them against the hazards associated with working with dangerous germs. They had also received many skin tests to detect immunity to different germs. Since 1950, the workers had received an average of more than 190 injections of 21 different vaccines, and 55 skin tests.

These 77 highly immunized workers were compared with 26 workers at the same laboratory who had not received special immunizations or been exposed to laboratory infections. At follow-up intervals of 10, 16 and 25 years, there were no important differences in history, physical examination or laboratory tests. There was no evidence of increased rates of cancer, immune disorders or death in the highly immunized group.

16 Why do vaccines contain formaldehyde, mercury, aluminum and other toxic chemicals?

Formaldehyde

Pertussis and inactivated polio vaccines are made from live bacteria or viruses that are killed with formaldehyde. Both tetanus and diphtheria toxins are inactivated with formaldehyde to make the toxoids. Following the inactivation process, purification of the vaccines removes almost all of the formaldehyde. The diphtheria, pertussis, tetanus, polio and Hib 5-in-1 vaccine contains less than 0.02% formaldehyde per dose, or less than 200 parts per million. This amount of formaldehyde is several hundred times lower than the amount known to cause harm to humans.

Mercury and thimerosal

Some vaccines used in Canada, the United States and other countries (diphtheria, tetanus, pertussis and hepatitis B vaccines) were once made with a preservative called thimerosal. No vaccine made in Canada since March 2001 for routine use in children contains thimerosal, and DTaP, polio and Hib vaccines have not contained this preservative since 1997-98.

Thimerosal contains mercury and is converted into ethylmercury in the body. Thimerosal is used to prevent bacterial contamination during production of the vaccine. The amount of thimerosal used in these vaccines is 0.01% per dose, or 100 parts per million. There is no scientific evidence that thimerosal has caused brain damage or other neurologic problems as a result of vaccination.

Aluminum

Several vaccines (such as diphtheria and tetanus toxoids, and hepatitis B vaccine) contain a complex salt of aluminum called alum. The amount of aluminum is less than 1 mg per dose. This amount of aluminum is not known to cause any harm to humans. Much larger quantities of aluminum salts are taken and absorbed into the body in the form of antacids (e.g., 200–400 mg of aluminum hydroxide per tablet) without any serious side effects.

Antibiotics

Some vaccines contain trace amounts of antibiotics used during the manufacturing process. The purpose of the antibiotics is to prevent bacterial contamination of the tissue culture cells in which the viruses are grown. Measles, mumps and rubella (MMR) vaccine and inactivated polio vaccine (IPV) each contain less than 25 micrograms of neomycin per dose (less than 0.000025 g).

17 Do vaccines contain blood, serum, animal tissue or fetal tissue?

No vaccine contains human blood or serum. Trace amounts of human albumin (a protein fractionated from whole blood) are used as a stabilizer in rabies vaccine and others. No vaccine contains animal or human cells. Viral vaccines are *grown* in cells derived from animals (chick embryo or monkey cells) or humans (fetal cells). At certain stages of production, calf serum may be added to fluid in which the cells are growing. (Calf serum is necessary for proper growth of cells in the test tube.)

During purification of the vaccine, *all* calf serum and *all* cells (animal or human) are removed. Trace amounts of some proteins from the cells may remain in the vaccine.

18 Don't some vaccines contain brain tissue, which can cause mad cow disease?

No. The only vaccine that ever contained brain tissue was the original rabies vaccine, which contained rabbit brain tissue. That vaccine is no longer used in Canada or the United States.

19 Can mercury in vaccines cause brain damage, retardation, autism, attention deficit disorder or learning disorders?

The issue of the potential toxicity of mercury in some vaccines has caused a great deal of discussion in the United States recently. Mercury was present in some vaccines in the form of thimerosal. Thimerosal is an organic mercury compound that has been used as a preservative in some vaccines and other medications since the 1930s. Thimerosal is *not* methylmercury. Methylmercury is a different compound, one that is known to cause brain damage.

Thimerosal

Thimerosal is used to prevent the growth of bacteria and fungi in multidose vials of vaccines. If such contamination occurred, it could cause serious infections in recipients of the vaccine. Thimerosal is also used as an inactivating or antibacterial agent in the manufacturing process for some vaccines. Such use contributes little to the final concentration of thimerosal in vaccines.

In the body, thimerosal is metabolized to ethylmercury (an organic compound) and thiosalicylate (a non-toxic substance). Ethylmercury is, therefore, the potential toxic substance. In 1999, the U.S. Federal Drug Administration determined that in following the recommended vaccination schedules in the United States, infants might be exposed to a total dose of ethylmercury that exceeded some federal safety guidelines established for ingestion of methylmercury. The safety guidelines were established for methylmercury because this compound is known to cause severe brain and nerve damage when toxic amounts are ingested. Much less is known about the toxicity of ethylmercury in humans.

Thimerosal in vaccines

Thimerosal is no longer a component of vaccines used in Canada for routine immunization of children. Even before it was discontinued though, there was much less use of thimerosal in Canadian vaccines than in American ones:

- Canada used inactivated polio vaccine (IPV) while the United States used oral polio vaccine (OPV). Combination vaccines that include IPV (such as DPT/IPV, DTaP/IPV) have never contained thimerosal. Thimerosal cannot be used with IPV-containing vaccines because it reduces the potency of the polio vaccine. The preservative used in these vaccines in Canada is phenoxyethanol — an alcohol compound that does not contain any mercury.
- DPT and DTaP vaccines made in the United States also used to contain thimerosal.

Expert committee conclusions

An expert committee of the Institute of Medicine in the United States recently reviewed all published and unpublished scientific evidence on the potential toxicity of thimerosal in vaccines. The committee came to the following conclusions based on the available scientific evidence:

- Low doses of thimerosal have not been shown to damage the nervous system in humans.
- Low doses of methylmercury have been shown to cause damage to the nervous system of fetuses; the damage resulted from exposure of the fetus to the compound before birth, not as a result of postnatal exposure.
- The toxicological information regarding ethylmercury, particularly at low doses, is limited.
- Thimerosal exposure from vaccines has not been proven to result in mercury levels known to be toxic in humans.
- Signs and symptoms of brain damage caused by mercury are not identical to those of autism, attention deficit hyperactivity disorder (ADHD), or speech or language delay.
- Autism is thought primarily to originate from prenatal injury to the fetus; exposure to ethylmercury has not been shown to cause any of the damage associated with autism.
- High-dose thimerosal exposure can cause neurological damage, but these doses are much higher than those observed in infants after vaccination with thimerosal-containing vaccines.

Vaccines today

There is no evidence that the presence of thimerosal in vaccines given appropriately has caused brain damage in any child. Newer production methods and availability of alternative preservatives have resulted in the discontinuation of use of thimerosal in vaccines used in infants in North America. Since it is no longer necessary, thimerosal has been removed from most vaccines on the principle that there should be no unnecessary substances in vaccines.

As of March 2001, all vaccines for routine immunization of children in Canada and the United States are produced *without* thimerosal. It is still used in certain vaccines that are *not* given to young infants, such as influenza vaccine.

Vaccines that contained thimerosal *before* March 2001

Canada	United States
• Hepatitis B	• DPT
• Influenza	• DTaP
• Hib	• Hepatitis B
• Meningococcal polysaccharide	• Influenza
	• Hib
	• Meningococcal polysaccharide

---

20 Can vaccines cause seizures?

Yes, indirectly. Vaccines can cause fever, and fever can cause convulsions. Therefore, vaccine-induced fever can cause convulsions, particularly in children who are susceptible (children whose parents or siblings have had convulsions are more likely to have a convulsion than those with no such history). Fever-related seizures are known as febrile seizures or convulsions.

Fever from any cause triggers a convulsion in about 3% of healthy young children. Fever is the most common cause of seizures or convulsions in infants between 6 months and 6 years of age. Febrile seizures *do not* cause brain damage.

21 Can pertussis vaccine cause brain damage?

The original pertussis vaccine made from killed bacteria was sometimes blamed for causing brain damage in infants and young children. A review of all of the scientific evidence carried out by the Institute of Medicine in the United States found that there is *no* proof that pertussis vaccine causes brain damage.

Studies

Four American studies were carried out involving more than 415,000 children who had received nearly 1 million doses of pertussis vaccine. The studies failed to find a single case of acute illness involving the brain, other than reports of convulsions (seizures) associated with fever. Such convulsions *do not* cause permanent damage. [See Question 20 for more information about convulsions.]

A study in the United Kingdom was also unable to find a single case of permanent brain damage that was clearly the result of vaccination. If brain damage does occur after vaccination, it is *extremely* rare.

When the recommended age for vaccination with pertussis vaccine was lowered in Denmark (from 5 months to 5 weeks) and raised in Japan (from 2 months to 2 years), there was no change in the age of onset of neurologic disease in infants.

Why then, has pertussis vaccine and almost every other vaccine been blamed for causing brain damage?

Temporal association

Vaccination is a very common and recognizable event in the first 6 months of life of most infants. Brain abnormalities, on the other hand, are uncommon and often unrecognizable in the first 6 months of life.

Most infants who have malformations of the brain or who suffer brain damage before birth or during labour and delivery appear to be normal for the first few months of life because the brain is not fully developed. Many babies are 4 to 6 months of age or more before it becomes clear that something is wrong with their development.

The diagnosis of cerebral palsy, mental retardation or developmental delay can usually not be made until the infant is several months old. By this time, the baby has already received one or more vaccinations, often with minor side effects such as fever, crying and fussiness. Since the infant appeared to be normal until the vaccine was given, the vaccine is blamed. [See Chapter 2 for a discussion of temporal association and cause and effect.]

The following facts make it extremely unlikely that pertussis vaccine can cause brain damage:
- Acute illness involving the brain has not been shown to be more common after vaccination than at any other time (except for febrile or fever-induced convulsions, which do not cause brain damage).
- Studies of large numbers of children have found that brain damage after vaccination is very rare, if it occurs at all.
- In searching for a link between brain damage and pertussis vaccine, no pattern of symptoms or abnormalities of laboratory tests have been found, and upon examination of the brain after death, no findings have been described that would establish pertussis vaccine as the cause of brain trauma.
- The damage in the brains of children who die of natural pertussis is caused by lack of oxygen and bleeding from small blood vessels as a result of severe coughing spells, not as a result of a toxin from the bacteria.
- No plausible mechanism has been found by which pertussis vaccination could cause brain damage.

22 Can measles vaccine or MMR vaccine cause autism or other developmental disorders?

The answer is no. However, some people believe otherwise because of the theory proposed by a British physician named Dr. Andrew Wakefield. In 1998, he described 12 children who he claimed had a new and unique form of bowel disease. Most of the children also were said to have autism, although that diagnosis was not confirmed. He claimed that symptoms of autism in these children developed soon after immunization with measles, mumps and rubella (MMR) vaccine.

Dr. Wakefield proposed the following theory in which he linked measles vaccine and autism:
1. MMR vaccine may produce damage to the bowel.
2. The bowel damage leads to either
   - impaired absorption of vitamins or micronutrients, or
   - an increase in intestinal absorption of intact proteins.
3. Either state leads to the formation of autoantibodies (antibodies that attack tissues in the body) that damage the brain.

There is *no* scientific evidence to support this theory. His original study had several important defects. Many studies have been performed following publication of his claims. These studies have attempted to answer the following questions:

1. Do symptoms of autism develop in children following immunization with MMR?

A large study of children with autism in England found that there was *no* association between the date at which MMR was given and the date when parents first became concerned about abnormal behaviour in their child.

Another study of 463 children with autism who were born in London between 1979 and 1998 found no change over this time period in the proportions of children with sudden regression of development or with bowel symptoms following the introduction of MMR vaccination in 1988. There were no differences in rates of bowel symptoms or regression in children who received MMR before their parents became concerned about their development compared with the rates in children who received MMR after the onset of autism or in children who did not receive the vaccine.

2. Has the frequency of autism increased since MMR was introduced?

The frequency of autism in the United States *appears* to have increased in recent years. However, this increase occurred long after MMR vaccine was introduced. No increase in autism rates was observed following the introduction of MMR vaccine in Canada, the United States, Europe or Japan. A separate Swedish study found no difference in the frequency of autism in children born before and after the introduction of MMR vaccine in Sweden.

What, then, could explain the rise in autism rates in some parts of the world? The most logical explanation is a change in the way the condition is assessed. Since 1990, there have been major changes in the criteria used to make the diagnosis of autism. Such changes have broadened the scope of the disorder to include many children with milder and atypical forms of autism. There is also much greater public awareness of autism and more parents are seeking help for their children.

3. Is there a relationship between the MMR vaccination rate and the autism rate?

In the United Kingdom, autism rates increased almost fourfold in boys who were born between 1988 and 1993. It would be logical that if there were a link between MMR vaccine and autism, the rates of both (autism and vaccination) would rise proportionately. But during this period, the MMR vaccination rate did not change, remaining steady at over 95%. And the rates of MMR vaccination were the same in children with and without autism.

In California, between 1980 and 1994, the number of children with autism enrolled in State Developmental Services programs increased 373%, while the MMR vaccination rate increased only 14%.

Conclusion

All published and unpublished evidence concerning MMR vaccine and autism has been reviewed independently by expert committees of the Institute of Medicine of the National Academy of Sciences in the United States and of the American Academy of Pediatrics. Both groups concluded that *there is no scientific evidence to support the theory that MMR causes autism or autistic spectrum disorders or inflammatory bowel disease.* [See Question 24 regarding unfounded theories on links between measles vaccine and inflammatory bowel disease.]

Dr. Wakefield recommended that it would be safer to give children measles vaccine, mumps vaccine and rubella vaccine as single vaccines at different times rather than as the combined MMR vaccine. In addition to the absence of any arguments or evidence to support his idea, there is no research confirming the proper sequence of or interval between vaccines given separately. There is also no information on the safety of the three vaccines given separately as a series of shots. There is no biologically plausible reason to think that separate vaccines would be safer or more effective than the combined vaccine.

23 Can vaccination cause cancer?

Cancer is relatively uncommon in children, affecting about 1 in 10,000 children under 15 years old. But because of the marked decline in death caused by infections that used to rank No. 1 (e.g., diphtheria, pertussis), cancer now is the second most common cause of death in children. (Accidents are No. 1.) There has been no significant increase in leukemia or other cancers in children since the start of routine vaccination in the 1940s. While it is difficult to prove that immunization never causes cancer, there is no scientific evidence of a link between the two. [See Chapter 2 for a discussion of cause and effect.]

However, vaccination can prevent cancer, indirectly. Persons infected with hepatitis B virus are over 40 times more likely to develop cancer of the liver compared with those not infected. The vaccine prevents infection with hepatitis B virus and this, in turn, prevents the liver cancer. Routine immunization of all infants in Taiwan has been shown to prevent infection with hepatitis B and to prevent liver cancer caused by hepatitis B.

24 Can vaccines cause MS, chronic fatigue syndrome or Crohn's disease?

Multiple sclerosis

There are more cases of multiple sclerosis (MS) today than 30 or more years ago. The reasons for this increase are: earlier and improved methods of diagnosis, improved treatment and longer survival of MS patients. The cause of MS is not yet known. There is some evidence suggesting that infection in childhood might play a role in the development of this disease. There is no evidence that immunization causes MS. In particular, hepatitis B and influenza vaccines have been shown to have no effect on symptoms or on rate of progression of symptoms in patients with MS.

Chronic fatigue syndrome

The cause of chronic fatigue syndrome is not known. Some opponents of vaccination have alleged that hepatitis B vaccination causes this illness. However, studies comparing vaccinated and unvaccinated adults did not show any increased risk of chronic fatigue syndrome after vaccination.

Other conditions

There are many other conditions for which causes are not yet known, such as **rheumatoid arthritis, Crohn's disease, ulcerative colitis and lupus erythromatosus (SLE).** Since most persons with these disorders were vaccinated in childhood, it is easy to blame the vaccine when no other cause can be found. However, there is no evidence to prove that these conditions are caused by vaccination.

Crohn's disease

Based on his findings in one recent study, Dr. Wakefield claimed that Crohn's disease (a chronic inflammation of the small intestines, of unknown causes) was more common in young adults who had received measles vaccine than in unvaccinated adults. The same researcher also claimed to have found genetic material of measles virus in samples of intestinal tissue from patients with Crohn's disease.

Additional studies have failed to find any association between measles vaccination and Crohn's disease or any other form of inflammatory bowel disease. Moreover, two other laboratories failed to confirm the claim that measles virus is present in samples of inflamed tissue from patients with Crohn's disease.

25 Can immunization cause SIDS?

There is *no* scientific evidence that immunization causes sudden infant death syndrome (SIDS). Claims have been made that babies are dying of SIDS following vaccination. However, the number of deaths after vaccination is no greater than would be expected by chance alone. Most cases of SIDS occur in infants less than 6 months of age. This is the same period during which babies are vaccinated. Therefore, the probability of the two events (vaccination and SIDS) occurring within a short time is extremely high (a temporal association).

Several large studies have found that there is no association between vaccination and SIDS. In fact, all of the studies found that babies who died of SIDS were less likely to have been vaccinated recently than were the babies in the control group (babies chosen to match the babies who died of SIDS, according to factors such as age, sex and weight to make comparisons).

In Canada, the United States, Australia, New Zealand and other countries that have used educational campaigns to teach parents to put their infants to sleep on their backs, there has been a huge drop in the SIDS rate. At the same time, immunization rates have increased in these countries.

26 Can vaccines cause Type I diabetes?

There is *no* scientific evidence that any vaccines increase the risk of Type I diabetes in humans or animals.

Type I diabetes, formerly known as juvenile or insulin-dependent diabetes, occurs primarily in children, but individuals of all ages can develop the disease. Most cases of Type I diabetes are caused by an autoimmune process. Autoimmunity occurs when an immune system develops antibodies and other immune responses directed against one or more organs in the body. Such autoimmune responses can cause damage to the organs involved.

Most persons have antibodies to islet cell antigens, even before Type I diabetes develops. The islet cells are the cells in the pancreas that make insulin. Persons with islet cell antibodies are at increased risk of developing Type I diabetes. The pancreas of persons with Type I diabetes shows damage consistent with autoimmune destruction of islet cells.

The following scientific observations lead to the conclusion that there is *no* relationship between vaccination and Type I diabetes:
• The incidence of Type I diabetes has increased in many countries. However such increases have not been associated with the introduction of any new childhood vaccines.
• There are no studies that reveal any significant differences in vaccination rates of children with Type I diabetes compared with the rates of healthy children without diabetes.

- Vaccination rates are the same for children at high risk for Type I diabetes who develop antibodies to islet cell antigens and children who do not develop antibodies.
- Studies in mice genetically predisposed to develop Type I diabetes show no effect of vaccines on the onset of the disorder.

27 Can vaccines cause asthma and other kinds of allergic disease?

There are certainly many anecdotes published claiming that asthma, eczema or some other kind of allergy developed after vaccination. However, recent studies have shown that immunization does not increase the frequency of asthma and other allergic diseases in children. For example, a large international study analyzed immunization rates and rates of asthma and other allergic diseases. Researchers obtained rates for 6- and 7-year-olds from 91 centres in 38 countries, and for 13- and 14-years-olds from 99 centres in 41 countries. They found no correlation between immunization rates and asthma/allergy rates.

28 Don't infections like measles stimulate the immune system and lead to better overall health?

In the 1980s, 180 Swiss naturopaths and homeopaths claimed that infection with measles in childhood is very important because it helps the immune system to develop in a natural and healthy way. They claimed that measles vaccine does not provide the same kind of stimulation and will weaken the immune strength of the population.

But it is *not* true that infection with measles is needed for normal development of the immune system. No infection acts as a general stimulus to the immune system. There is no scientific evidence that infection with measles or any other germ is necessary or important for natural and healthy development of the immune system.

No prerequisites for "normal" development

In fact, what we know of measles makes it extremely unlikely that measles plays any role whatsoever in the normal development — if there is such a thing — of the human immune system. For example, we know that measles cannot survive among small groups of people, like those living in isolated tribes in the Amazon rain forest or on islands. Yet such people have perfectly normal immune systems.

For most of human history, we were without measles. It became common only after the development of agriculture and the rise of cities, as measles thrives only in highly populated areas. Because the infection is so contagious, it spreads rapidly to all susceptible members of a group. In a city, there are always new, susceptible individuals entering the group as a result of large numbers of births. In a small tribe on an island, however, the measles virus would quickly die out.

Measles suppresses the immune system

Natural infection with measles does not provide a general form of stimulation of the immune system. It stimulates immunity to measles only. In fact, measles infection results in marked suppression of many parts of the immune system, a state that lasts several months. During this time, the child is more susceptible to a number of other infections. This suppression of the immune system caused by measles actually leads to the high rate of other infections that complicate measles.

Thus, measles does nothing good to the immune system other than stimulate immunity to measles. Infection with measles not only results in a severe illness, which has a high rate of complications and general impairment of health, but it also suppresses the immune system for several months.

Other infections may produce similar types of immune suppression, but to a lesser degree than measles.

29 Is vaccination safer when my child is older rather than at 2 months of age?

There is no evidence that side effects from vaccination are more common in younger infants. The purpose of starting vaccination at 2 months of age is to protect the child against pertussis and Hib disease as early in life as possible. Complications and deaths from pertussis are most common in infants less than 6 months of age. And infants *can* respond to vaccination at a very young age [see Question 15].

The combination product used in Canada containing diphtheria and tetanus toxoids, and acellular pertussis, inactivated polio and Hib vaccines minimizes the number of injections given to each child. Giving these vaccines at the same time *does not* increase the rate of side effects. The protection achieved by the combined vaccine is as great as giving the vaccines as separate injections.

30 Who should not be vaccinated?

In general, anyone who has had anaphylaxis or any other severe allergic reaction after a vaccine should not be vaccinated again until the cause of the reaction has been determined. Anaphylaxis is a severe allergic reaction in which the person goes into shock and has difficulty breathing. It usually occurs within minutes of exposure to the source of the allergy.

Anyone with a serious disorder of the immune system should not receive live virus vaccines such as oral polio, measles, mumps and rubella and varicella vaccines. This includes persons with severe congenital immune deficiency disorders, persons receiving chemotherapy for cancer, persons who have had a bone marrow or other organ transplant, and persons receiving high doses of steroids. [See Table 17.3 at the end of this Chapter.]

31 When should vaccination be delayed?

Severe illness at the scheduled time of vaccination warrants a delay until the child has recovered. Vaccination should *not* be delayed because of minor illnesses such as colds, coughs or low-grade fevers (39–39.5°C/102–103°F). Children with minor illnesses of this sort respond normally to vaccination and have no added side effects.

In the past, pertussis vaccination has often been deferred in children with progressive or changing neurologic conditions. Such conditions include tuberous sclerosis, recurrent convulsions that are not prevented by medication, and neurodegenerative diseases. Research reveals that there is no need to defer the pertussis vaccine in such children. If it is withheld for some reason, diphtheria and tetanus toxoids can still be administered without the pertussis vaccine.

Anyone who has received immune globulin (made from the plasma of blood donors) by injection into muscle or a vein should not receive measles, mumps or rubella vaccine for 3 months or more, depending on the dose of immune globulin. The antibodies in this blood product can interfere with establishment of immunity after vaccination. [See Table 17.3 at the end of this Chapter.]

32 What conditions are not reasons to delay vaccination?

Sometimes it is necessary to delay vaccination, as discussed in the previous question. However, it is *not* necessary to delay vaccination for the following reasons:

- minor infections such as colds, coughs or diarrhea (assuming there is no serious change in the child's behaviour);
- high fever (40°C/104°F or higher) after a previous dose of vaccine;
- prolonged inconsolable crying (for more than 3 hours) after a previous dose of vaccine;
- large local reactions (more than 5 cm) after a previous dose of vaccine;
- history of convulsions, with or without fever;
- a hypotonic-hyporesponsive episode (HHE) [see Chapter 5, under *Possible side effects of pertussis vaccine*, for details] following a previous vaccination — such episodes have not been shown to cause permanent damage of any kind and do not recur with subsequent vaccinations;
- active allergy, asthma or eczema;
- allergy to eggs;
- current antibiotic treatment;
- infant born prematurely;
- recent exposure to a minor infection (such as a cold — again, assuming there is no serious change in the child's behaviour);
- family history of sudden infant death syndrome (SIDS);
- progressive or changing neurologic conditions [see Question 31 for more detail];
- breastfeeding (both the breastfeeding woman and breastfed baby can safely be vaccinated);
- child's mother is pregnant.

TABLE 17.3

Contraindications to routine childhood vaccines

VACCINE	TRUE CONTRAINDICATION	PRECAUTIONS†	NOT A CONTRAINDICATION
All vaccines	Anaphylaxis after previous dose of vaccine or to any component of the vaccine.	Moderate or severe acute illness with or without fever.	Severe local reaction to previous dose of vaccine. Mild cold or acute illness. Antibiotic treatment. Prematurity at birth. Personal or family history of allergy.
DTaP	Anaphylaxis after previous dose of vaccine.	Hypotonic-hyporesponsive hyporesponsive episode (HHE) after previous dose of vaccine.	High fever, convulsions, inconsolable crying, encephalopathy or HHE after previous doses of vaccine. Family history of SIDS or of convulsions.
IPV	Anaphylaxis after previous dose of vaccine. Allergy to neomycin.		
MMR	Anaphylaxis after previous dose of vaccine. Pregnancy.	Recent injection of immune globulin. Severe allergy to gelatin (administer with great caution). Immunosuppression from disease or medical treatment.	TB or positive TB skin test. Egg allergy.
Hib, MC, PC	Anaphylaxis after previous dose of vaccine.		History of disease caused by Hib, MC or PC.
Hepatitis B	Anaphylaxis after previous dose of vaccine.		Pregnancy.
Influenza	Anaphylaxis after eating eggs.		Pregnancy.
Varicella	Anaphylaxis after previous dose of vaccine. Pregnancy	Immunosuppression from disease or medical treatment.	

DTaP: diphtheria and tetanus toxoids, acellular pertussis vaccine
IPV: inactivated polio vaccine
MMR: measles, mumps and rubella vaccine
Hib: *Haemophilus influenzae* type b vaccine; MC: meningococcal vaccine; PC: pneumococcal vaccine
Varicella: chickenpox vaccine
† Precautions are not contraindications, but events or conditions to be considered in determining if the benefits of vaccine outweigh the risks.

Glossary
acute illness: common cold, acute diarrhea
anaphylaxis: severe allergic reaction leading to one or more of the following: shock, facial swelling, swelling of eyelids, wheezing, difficulty breathing
convulsions: seizure
encephalopathy: severe disturbance of brain function with seizures and changes in state of consciousness, coma
hypotonic-hyporesponsive episode (HHE): sudden paleness, decreased responsiveness, loss of muscle tone or floppiness
immune globulin: protein solution prepared from plasma (blood) containing a high concentration of antibodies
immunosuppression: depression of immune system responses caused by disease (e.g., leukemia, cancer, HIV/AIDS) or by treatment (e.g., cancer chemotherapy, high doses of steroids)
local reaction: redness, swelling, pain, and/or tenderness at site of injection
neomycin: antibiotic used during growth of viruses in tissue culture
TB: tuberculosis

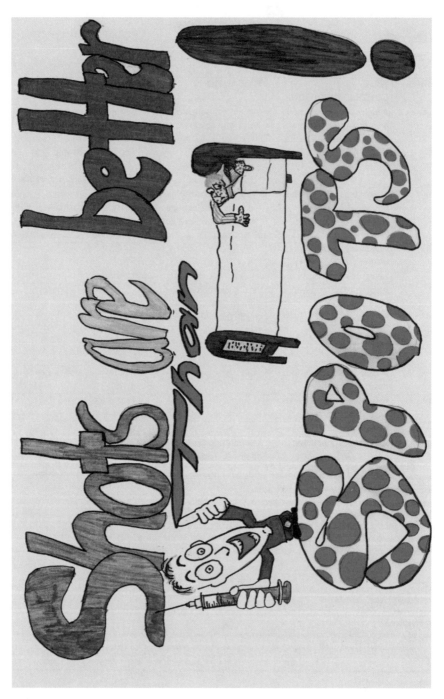

Andrew Newman, Fergus, Ontario

CHAPTER 18

Resources

Misinformation About Vaccines

The Internet offers access to a wealth of information about vaccines, diseases and immunization. But it also houses a wealth of misinformation. It would be wonderful if only factual, truthful information was posted on the Internet. But this is not the case. No one regulates the validity of information that is available to millions of people.

So it is up to you, the consumer, to assess the validity of the information. This chapter will help you to determine whether the source of your information is credible and whether the information itself is reliable. (The tips provided can be useful in evaluating any vaccine-related information.)

Later in the chapter, you'll find many credible sources to consult if you're looking for answers to questions or wanting to know more about what you have read in this book.

Tips on Evaluating Information

In your search for information about vaccines, you will probably come across sources you're not sure about. The questions below will help you judge whether or not the information is reliable. These questions were written specifically for information obtained from the Internet; but they are useful to ask of any media source, including newspapers, magazines, radio, tabloids, pamphlets or books.

What is the source of the information?
• The website should clearly identify the person or organization that produced it.
• The site should provide a way to contact the provider of information.

Has the medical information been reviewed by scientific experts?
• If yes, the experts should be identified, including their credentials (degrees, positions, etc.).

Is there a date indicating when the information was last revised?
• If yes, is it current?

Is there scientific evidence to support the claims?
• If yes, the site should provide sources (e.g., articles from medical journals) for the scientific evidence (e.g., studies, reports, statistics).

Is the site certified by the Health On the Net Foundation?
• Health On the Net (HON) Foundation is a Swiss not-for-profit organization working to help Internet users find useful and reliable

on-line medical information. HON has developed a set of guidelines for health sites. Sites that meet the criteria can use the HON seal to show they follow the code of conduct. The HON site (www.hon.ch) also has a checklist to help users judge whether a given site would meet the criteria.

Anti-vaccination websites. A recent study of 22 websites that oppose vaccination found that the sites shared a number of features (*Journal of American Medical Association*, 2002, vol. 287, pp. 3245–8).
- They made the same false claims about vaccines.
- They all had links to other anti-vaccination sites.
- Many promoted alternative systems of health care — such as homeopathy, naturopathy and chiropractic — as being superior to vaccination.
- More than half provided anecdotes about children who had allegedly been damaged by vaccines.

False claims made on anti-vaccination websites include the following:
- Vaccines cause illnesses whose causes are unknown, such as autism (from MMR and/or DTaP), SIDS, immune dysfunction, diabetes, seizures, brain damage, attention deficit disorder, antisocial behaviour, asthma, allergy (100% of sites).
- Vaccines erode immunity or harm the immune system (95% of sites).
- Vaccine producers or government regulators are responsible for an underreporting of adverse reactions because they cover up the truth about such events (95% of sites).
- Vaccine policy is motivated by profit: manufacturers make enormous profits on vaccines, which influences vaccine recommendations and promotes cover up of reactions (91% of sites).
- Vaccines are ineffective or produce only temporary immunity (82% of sites).
- Compulsory vaccination violates civil rights (77% of sites).
- Rates of disease declined prior to the use of vaccines due to improved nutrition (73% of sites).

- Lots of vaccines cause severe reactions (55% of sites).
- There is an increased risk of reactions from multiple simultaneous vaccines (50% of sites).
- Homeopathy, naturopathy, alternative medicine and breastfeeding enhance immunity better than vaccines.

If you are in doubt about any information you read or hear, discuss it with your health-care professional.

Credible Sites† and Resources

Canadian Sites

Canadian Paediatric Society

www.cps.ca

This is the main website for the Canadian Paediatric Society (CPS). It includes all position statements published by the Infectious Diseases and Immunization Committee. It's recommended for health care professionals and others who want detailed, scientific information about vaccines and vaccine-preventable diseases. The CPS website also includes information about IMPACT, a vaccine surveillance program, and about the Canadian Paediatric Surveillance Program (CPSP), a rare-disease surveillance program [see Chapter 2 for more information].

www.caringforkids.cps.ca

Caring for Kids is a website for parents, developed and maintained by the CPS. It contains easy-to-read documents on vaccines and immunization, as well as many other pages on children's health, safety, growth and development.

Health Canada, Division of Immunization

www.hc-sc.gc.ca/hpb/lcdc/bid/di/index.html

Here you'll find information and recommendations from the National Advisory Committee on Immunization, as well as an on-line version of the *Canadian Immunization Guide*.

Canadian Immunization Awareness Program
www.immunize.cpha.ca

The Canadian Immunization Awareness Program (CIAP) is
a coalition of health and medical groups, managed through the
Canadian Public Health Association (CPHA). Its website
includes a resources section that is updated regularly.

Meningitis Research Foundation of Canada
www.meningitis.ca

This site provides information about meningitis, including a
description of the disease and how it is spread, treated and
prevented.

American Sites

American Academy of Pediatrics
www.aap.org

The American Academy of Pediatrics (AAP) website includes
the organization's policy statements on immunization, as well as
other issues.

www.cispimmunize.org

The Childhood Immunization Support Program (CISP) was
started by the AAP, in partnership with the Centers for Disease
Control and Prevention. CISP supports U.S. paediatricians
delivering immunization and provides education and resources
on immunization and related issues. The CISP website features
videos of immunizations as well as pages devoted to research,
Q&As for families, and resources for health care providers, to
name a few.

Centers for Disease Control and Prevention
www.cdc.gov

The Centers for Disease Control and Prevention (CDC) is the
U.S. federal public health agency. You can search through its
massive website using a search engine or an alphabetical menu
of health topics.

www.cdc.gov/ncidod
The National Center for Infectious Diseases (NCID) provides in-depth information on infectious diseases, including vaccine-preventable diseases, through a searchable index.

www.cdc.gov/nip
The CDC's National Immunization Program has many resources for parents, including a booklet called *Parents Guide to Childhood Immunization*,* which contains straightforward information on vaccine-preventable diseases: www.cdc.gov/nip/publications/ Parents-Guide/default.htm. Other useful items include the current U.S. immunization schedules, information on vaccine safety, how to report vaccine-related side effects, and a list of reliable resources.

www.cdc.gov.nip/publications
This section contains publications and fact sheets for the public, as well as the recommendations of the Advisory Committee on Immunization Practices of the U.S. Public Health Services and Vaccine Information Statements for parents.

www.cdc.gov/nip/vacsafe
This section concentrates on vaccine safety issues.

Children's Vaccine Program
www.childrensvaccine.org
The focus of the Children's Vaccine Program, a partnership of U.S. and international groups, is vaccination for children worldwide.

Immunization Action Coalition
www.immunize.org
While this site is most suited to health professionals, it contains much useful information for parents. It includes personal accounts of people affected by vaccine-preventable diseases. It also provides

a link to a discussion on vaccine myths, www.immunize.org/catg.d/
4038myth.htm, and to a directory of resources, www.immunize.org/
resources/contents.htm

Institute for Vaccine Safety, Johns Hopkins University
www.vaccinesafety.edu
This site includes information on vaccines and the diseases they
prevent and commentaries on current vaccine safety issues.

Institute of Medicine (IOM)
**www.iom.edu/iom/iomhome.nsf/Pages/immunization+
safety+review**
The Institute of Medicine (IOM) site contains the reports of
the Immunization Safety Review Committee, including one on
MMR and autism and another on thimerosal in vaccines.

National Network for Immunization Information
www.immunizationinfo.org
National Network for Immunization Information (NNii) is a
partnership of several U.S. medical organizations, including the
Infectious Diseases Society of America, the Pediatric Infectious
Diseases Society and the American Academy of Pediatrics. It
publishes *Immunization Newsbriefs* — which can be read on-line
or as an e-mail newsletter — three times a week to highlight
vaccine issues in the news. The site has a searchable database
on vaccine-preventable diseases, as well as information on
vaccine development and safety, guidelines on evaluating on-
line information, and an extensive annotated list of websites.
The NNii Resource Kit, *Communicating with Patients about
Immunization,** is available in a downloadable PDF format.

National Partnership for Immunization
www.partnersforimmunization.org
National Partnership for Immunization (NPI) is a joint partnership of the National Healthy Mothers, Healthy Babies Coalition

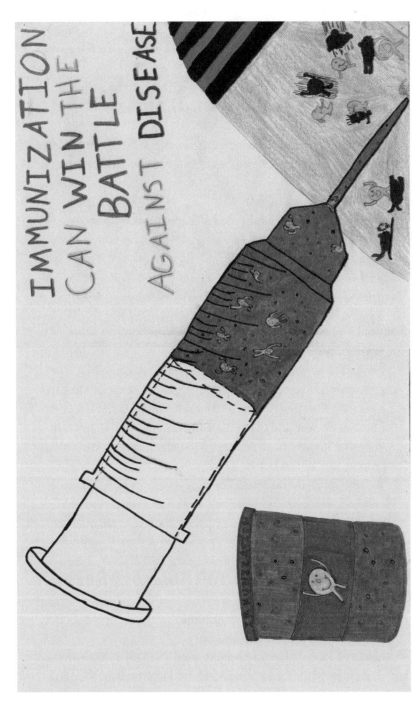

Miranda Doetzel, Macklin, Saskatchewan

and the National Foundation for Infectious Diseases. NPI has published a *Reference Guide for Vaccines and Vaccine Safety,** which is a comprehensive summary of the scientific evidence for vaccination: www.partnersforimmunization.org/guidebook.html

Parents of Kids with Infectious Diseases
www.pkids.org
This site, known as PKIDS, contains information, articles, Q&As on immunization, and an "Ask the Experts" feature that allows users to e-mail their questions.

Vaccine Education Center at the Children's Hospital of Philadelphia
www.vaccine.chop.edu*
This site aims to provide complete, up-to-date and reliable vaccine information to parents and health professionals. It includes information on vaccine safety, how vaccines work, how they are made, who recommends them, when they should be given and why they are necessary.

Books

National Advisory Committee on Immunization, Health Canada. *Canadian Immunization Guide*, 6th edition (Ottawa: Canadian Medical Association), 2002.*

Offit, Paul A. and Bell, Louis M. *Vaccines: What Every Parent Should Know,* Revised edition (New York: IDG Books), 1999.

Pickering, Larry K., ed. *2000 Red Book: Report of the Committee on Infectious Diseases*, 25th edition (Elk Grove Village, IL: American Academy of Pediatrics), 2000.*

Plotkin, Stanley A., and Mortimer, Edward A., eds. *Vaccines*, 3rd edition. (Philadelphia, PA: WB Saunders Company), 1999.*

Fact Sheets

The Canadian Paediatric Society has prepared a series of fact sheets on childhood vaccines. They appear in Chapter 19.

The fact sheets have been designed for easy photocopying. People working in health care settings can reproduce them without permission.

* Indicates the resources used in the development of this book.

† Internet addresses cited throughout this book were current as of December 2002.

Fact Sheets on Childhood Vaccines

This chapter summarizes information on the diseases and vaccines that have been described in more detail in the preceding pages. Any questions you have about vaccines after reading this book should be answered by your doctor, public health nurse or local medical officer of health — *before* your child is vaccinated.

About this information

These fact sheets give you basic information about vaccines and the diseases they protect against. They should not be used as a substitute for the medical care and advice of your doctor. Treatment can vary based on individual facts and circumstances.

Health care professionals may reproduce these sheets without permission and share them with patients and their families.

Vaccines available in Canada, as of December 2002

VACCINE	BRAND NAMES	ABBREVIATION	TYPE OF VACCINE	MANUFACTURER	GIVEN BY
Diphtheria and tetanus toxoids and acellular pertussis	Tripacel	DTaP	Inactivated, purified bacterial products	Aventis Pasteur	Injection
Diphtheria and tetanus toxoids and acellular pertussis and inactivated polio vaccine	Quadracel	DTaP-IPV	Inactivated, purified bacterial products and killed virus	Aventis Pasteur	Injection
Diphtheria and tetanus toxoids and acellular pertussis and inactivated polio polio vaccine and *Haemophilus influenzae* type b conjugate vaccine	Pentacel	DTaP-IPV-Hib	Inactivated, purified bacterial products and killed virus	Aventis Pasteur	Injection
Diphtheria and tetanus toxoids, and inactivated polio vaccine paediatric formulation	na (not applicable)	DT-IPV	Inactivated, purified bacterial products and killed virus	Aventis Pasteur	Injection
Tetanus and diphtheria toxoids, adult formulation	na	Td	Inactivated, purified bacterial products	Aventis Pasteur	Injection
Tetanus and diphtheria toxoids, and inactivated polio vaccine, adult formulation	na	Td-IPV	Inactivated, purified bacterial products and killed virus	Aventis Pasteur	Injection
Tetanus and diphtheria toxoids, and acellular pertusis vaccine, adult formulation	Adacel	dTap	Inactivated, purified bacterial products	Aventis Pasteur	Injection
Haemophilus influenzae type b conjugate vaccine	Act-HIB HibTITER PedvaxHIB	PRP-T PRP-CRM PRP-OMP	Purified bacterial product	Aventis Pasteur Wyeth-Ayerst Merck Frosst	Injection
Measles-Mumps-Rubella vaccine	MMR-II Priorix	MMR	Live, attenuated virus	Merck Frosst GlaxoSmithKline	Injection
Chickenpox vaccine (Varicella)	Varivax II Varilrix	na (not applicable)	Live, attenuated virus	Merck Frosst GlaxoSmithKline	Injection
Meningococcal groups A/C/Y/W135 polysaccharide vaccine	Menomune	na	Purified bacterial products	Aventis Pasteur	Injection

VACCINE	BRAND NAMES	ABBREVIATION	TYPE OF VACCINE	MANUFACTURER	GIVEN BY
Meningococcal groups A and C polysaccharide vaccine	Mencevax AC Group A and C	na	Purified bacterial products	GlaxoSmithKline Aventis Pasteur	Injection
Meningococcal C conjugate vaccine	Menjugate NeisVac-C	na	Purified bacterial products	Merck Frosst Baxter/Shire Biologics	Injection
Pneumococcal polysaccharide vaccine	Pneumovax-23 Pneumo 23 Pnu-Imune 23	na	Purified bacterial products	Merck Frosst Aventis Pasteur Wyeth-Ayerst	Injection
Pneumococcal conjugate vaccine	Prevnar	na	Purified bacterial products	Wyeth-Ayerst	Injection
Hepatitis A vaccine	Havrix Vaqta Avaxim Paediatric Epaxal Berna	na	Inactivated virus	GlaxoSmithKline Merck Frosst Aventis Pasteur Swiss Serum and Vaccine Institute	Injection
Hepatitis B vaccine	Engerix-B Recombivax-HB	na	Purified viral protein	GlaxoSmithKline Merck Frosst	Injection
Hepatitis A/ Hepatitis B combined vaccine	Twinrix Twinrix Junior	na	Inactivated virus/purified viral protein	GlaxoSmithKline	Injection
Influenza vaccine	Fluzone Vaxigrip Fluviral	na	Inactivated split virus	Aventis Pasteur Aventis Pasteur Shire Biologics	Injection
Japanese encephalitis virus vaccine	JE-Vax	na	Inactivated virus	Biken/Aventis Pasteur	Injection
Typhoid vaccine	Vivotif Berna	na	Live, attenuated bacteria	Swiss Serum and Vaccine Institute	Oral
Typhoid vaccine	Typhim Vi Thypherix	na	Purified bacterial product	Aventis Pasteur GlaxoSmithKline	Injection
Yellow fever	YF-Vax	na	Live, attenuated virus	Aventis Pasteur	Injection

About this information

This fact sheet gives you basic information about vaccines and the diseases they protect against. It should not be used as a substitute for the medical care and advice of your doctor. Treatment can vary based on individual facts and circumstances. Ask your doctor any questions you have about the vaccine *before* your child is vaccinated.

Health care professionals may reproduce these sheets without permission and share them with patients and their families.

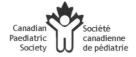

Canadian Paediatric Society

Société canadienne de pédiatrie

100–2204 Walkley Road, Ottawa, ON K1G 4G8 Tel.: (613) 526-9397 Fax: (613) 526-3332 www.caringforkids.cps.ca

5-in-1 Vaccine

You can protect your children from 5 diseases by giving them 1 easy shot. Other words for "shot" are needle, booster and vaccine. The 5-in-1 shot protects children against:
1. Diphtheria,
2. Tetanus,
3. Pertussis,
4. Polio, and
5. Hib.

In Canada, most children get the 5-in-1 shot when they are:
- 2 months old,
- 4 months old,
- 6 months old, and
- 18 months old.

Children get a booster of the 4-in-1 at 4 to 6 years of age. A booster of Hib vaccine is not needed again at this age in children who have already received the vaccine. The 4-in-1 shot protects against:
1. Diphtheria,
2. Tetanus,
3. Pertussis, and
4. Polio.

If you want to protect your children, you need to bring them back to get all their shots at the right time. Your doctor or nurse can give you a record book to help keep track of the shots. Ask for one.

What is diphtheria?
- It is an illness caused by germs (bacteria) that infect the nose, throat or skin.
- It causes serious problems with breathing. It can also cause heart failure and nerve damage for the rest of your life.
- Of every 10 people who get diphtheria, 1 will die from it. Babies who get it are even more likely to die.

What is tetanus?
- It is also called lockjaw.
- It is caused by germs (bacteria) that live in dirt and dust.
- When the tetanus germ gets into an open cut, poison from the germ can spread to nerves and then to muscles. Muscles may lock in one place or go into spasms (get very tight). This is very painful.
- The first muscles affected are the ones in the jaw. Your child may not be able to swallow or open his or her mouth. This is why tetanus is called lockjaw.
- If tetanus gets to the muscles that help your child breathe, your child can die very quickly.
- Children who survive tetanus may have long-lasting problems with speech, memory and thinking. Even if they have it once, they can still get it again.
- The tetanus shot protects both adults and children. Ask your doctor how you can get a tetanus shot so you can protect yourself, too.

What is pertussis?
- It is also called whooping cough. It used to kill many young children.
- It is caused by germs (bacteria) that get into the throat and lungs.
- Children may cough so long and so hard that they can't breathe.
- Babies with whooping cough may have fits (seizures) and go into a

coma. 1 out of 400 babies under a year old who gets whooping cough will end up with brain damage.

- Older children who get whooping cough will have 2 to 3 weeks of severe coughing spells. The disease can last from 6 to 12 weeks.

What is polio?

- It is a disease caused by 1 of 3 types of the polio virus. (A virus is a kind of germ that can make people sick.)
- Polio can cause fever, headache, vomiting (throwing up), strong muscle pain and muscles that won't move (are paralyzed). It can also make children very tired and cause stiffness in the neck and back.
- Some people with polio don't feel sick at all. Others are paralyzed (can't move their arms or legs) for the rest of their lives. Some people die.

What is Hib?

- Hib stands for *Haemophilus influenzae* type b. In spite of its name, it has nothing to do with the flu.
- Hib is the name of germs (bacteria) that can infect the fluid around the brain and spinal cord.

- Hib can cause a very serious disease called meningitis. Without treatment, all children who get this disease will die or suffer damage that lasts for the rest of their lives. Hib can also lead to other serious diseases that can kill.
- Even with treatment, about 1 in 20 children with Hib meningitis will die.
- About 1 in 3 children who survive Hib meningitis will have brain damage.

How safe is the 5-in-1 shot?

- It is very safe.
- The only children who should not get the 5-in-1 shot are those who had trouble breathing or had severe swelling of the skin or mouth shortly after receiving the shot before.
- With any vaccine, there may be some redness, swelling or pain at the place where the needle went into the arm or leg.
- Some children will have a fever after they get the shot. Ask your doctor what to give to control the fever or pain.
- If you have any questions about the 5-in-1 vaccine (DTap/IPV + Hib), ask your doctor.

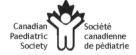

Canadian Paediatric Society   Société canadienne de pédiatrie

100–2204 Walkley Road, Ottawa, ON K1G 4G8 Tel.: (613) 526-9397 Fax: (613) 526-3332 www.caringforkids.cps.ca

MMR (Measles Mumps Rubella) Vaccine

You can protect your child from 3 diseases by giving them 1 easy vaccine called MMR. It protects children against:
1. Measles,
2. Mumps, and
3. Rubella

In Canada, children should get the MMR shot twice. They can get it when they are:
- 12 months old and 18 months old, *or*
- 12 months old and before they start school (between ages 4 and 6).

It is safe to give the second MMR shot 1 month after the first MMR shot.

If you are thinking about getting pregnant and did not have rubella (German measles) when you were younger, there are very good reasons why you should get the shot now. Read the section called *What about pregnant women and rubella?* later on in this fact sheet.

What is measles?
- It is a disease caused by a virus. A virus is a kind of germ that can make people sick.
- Sometimes it is called red measles (or rubeola) so it will not be confused with German measles (or rubella).
- Measles begins with a fever, runny nose, a cough and very red eyes. You may think your child has a cold.
- In a few days, a rash begins around the face and spreads to the chest, arms and legs. The eyes may hurt in bright light.
- Measles can cause an ear infection or pneumonia (a serious disease where fluid fills the lungs).

- Out of 1,000 children who get measles, 1 will also get a swelling of the brain called encephalitis. This can lead to fits (seizures), deafness, mental retardation or death.
- There is no treatment for measles.

How is measles spread?
It spreads quickly by sneezing and coughing. It is very easy to catch measles.

What is mumps?
- It is a disease caused by a virus. A virus is a kind of germ that can make people sick.
- Mumps is most common in children, although sometimes adults get it, too.
- Mumps causes fever, headache and swelling of the saliva glands (inside the mouth). This swelling is painful and makes the cheeks puff out.
- Sometimes, mumps can cause meningitis, a serious disease that infects the fluid around the brain and spinal cord.
- Mumps can cause deafness.
- In adults, mumps can affect a woman's eggs or a man's sperm. A man who gets mumps may become sterile (not able to have children). For both men and women, mumps can be very painful.

How is mumps spread?
It is spread by close contact between people. Sneezing and coughing can spread the disease.

What is rubella?
- It is also called German measles. Like red measles, rubella is caused by a

virus. A virus is a kind of germ that can make people sick.
- It is a milder disease than red measles. Children get a low fever and a mild cold. A rash may follow. Glands in the neck may swell up. The sickness lasts about 3 days.

How is rubella spread?
It is spread by close contact between people. Sneezing and coughing can spread the disease.

What about pregnant women and rubella?
- A pregnant woman who catches rubella during the first 5 months of pregnancy can pass the disease on to her baby (or fetus) while it is in the womb. The chances of this happening are very high. In 8 out of 10 cases where a pregnant woman has rubella in the first 5 months of pregnancy, the fetus will get rubella before it is born.
- If the fetus gets rubella during the first 12 weeks of pregnancy, it will likely be born with many physical problems. The baby may be blind, deaf or have heart damage.
- If the fetus gets rubella between 16 and 20 weeks of pregnancy, it will probably be born deaf.
- 1 out of 10 babies who are born with rubella will die during the first 12 months of life.

- There is no treatment for rubella in babies. The damage that happens to the fetus will last for the child's whole life.

What can you do?
- Before you get pregnant, have a simple blood test. It will tell you if you had rubella as a child.
- If the blood test shows you did *not* have rubella as a child, you should get the shot right away.
- Don't wait until you are pregnant. You should *not* have the MMR shot when you are pregnant.
- Speak to your doctor if you are planning to get pregnant.

How safe is the MMR vaccine?
- It is very safe. The only children who should not get the MMR shot are those who had trouble breathing *or* had severe swelling on the skin or in the mouth after their first shot.
- With any vaccine, there may be some redness, swelling, or pain at the place where the needle went into the arm or leg. Some children will have a fever and a rash. Some have joint pains that last a little while. Your doctor can tell you what to give to control the fever or pain.
- If you have questions about the MMR vaccine, ask your doctor.

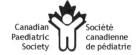

Canadian Paediatric Society
Société canadienne de pédiatrie

100–2204 Walkley Road, Ottawa, ON K1G 4G8 Tel.: (613) 526-9397 Fax: (613) 526-3332 www.caringforkids.cps.ca

Chickenpox Vaccine

You can protect your young child or teenager from chickenpox by making sure they get a simple shot. Other words for "shot" are needle, booster and vaccine.

In Canada:
- Children from 1 to 12 years of age get the shot once.
- Teens who are 13 to 19 years of age get 2 shots, 4 weeks apart.

Adults who have never had chickenpox should get the same number of shots as teens.

What is chickenpox?

It is an illness caused by the varicella-zoster virus. A virus is a kind of germ that can make people sick.

People with chickenpox get an itchy rash or spots on their skin. The spots are like small water blisters. Some people have only a few blisters; others can have as many as 500. These blisters dry up and form scabs in 4 or 5 days.

How is chickenpox spread?

Chickenpox spreads very quickly.
- It spreads from person to person through direct contact. You can get chickenpox if you touch a blister or the liquid from a blister. You can also get chickenpox if you touch the spit of a person who has chickenpox. The virus can get into your nose or mouth and make you sick also.
- It can also spread through the air, if you are near someone with chickenpox who is coughing or sneezing.
- A pregnant woman with chickenpox can pass it on to her baby before birth.
- Mothers with chickenpox can also give it to their newborn babies after birth.

How common is chickenpox?

Chickenpox is a very common sickness. Most people get chickenpox by the time they are 15 years old. In Canada, there are about 350,000 new cases each year among children and teens under 15 years of age.

Can chickenpox cause bigger problems?

- If the blisters get infected, you may end up with scars.
- In rare cases, the skin blisters can become infected with the same germs (tetanus) that cause infection after cuts and scrapes. This kind of infection can be very severe. It could even cause death.
- Children with chickenpox may get pneumonia (infection of the lungs) or have problems with other organs inside the body, such as the brain.
- Babies who get chickenpox from their mothers before birth can be born with birth defects. Some examples of these birth defects are

skin scars, eye problems, or arms and legs that are not fully formed.

- Chickenpox can be very severe or even life-threatening to newborn babies, adults and anyone who has a weak immune system.

Who should *not* have the chickenpox vaccine?

- Babies less than 1 year old.
- People with weak immune systems and people who are taking drugs to suppress their immune system. (Sometimes these people can get the vaccine, but they should talk to their doctor about this.)
- Women who are trying to get pregnant. They should talk to their doctor first.
- People who are allergic to or have had a bad reaction to something in the vaccine.
- People who have had chickenpox do not need to get the vaccine. They are most likely immune to it now.

If they do get the vaccine, it will not hurt them.

- Your doctor will question you to make sure it is okay for you to get the vaccine.

How safe is the chickenpox vaccine?

- It is very safe.
- With any vaccine, there may be some redness, swelling or pain at the place where the needle went into the arm or leg.
- Ask your doctor what you can do to control pain or swelling.
- Some people will get a very mild case of chickenpox 1 or 2 weeks after they get the vaccine. They will most likely have less than 50 spots.
- The chickenpox vaccine can be given at the same time as the MMR (Measles, Mumps, Rubella) vaccine.
- If you have any questions about the chickenpox vaccine, ask your doctor.

© CPS, December 2002

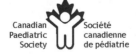

Canadian Paediatric Society

Société canadienne de pédiatrie

100–2204 Walkley Road, Ottawa, ON K1G 4G8 Tel.: (613) 526-9397 Fax: (613) 526-3332 www.caringforkids.cps.ca

Pneumococcal Vaccine

What is pneumococcal disease?

- Pneumococcal infections are caused by a germ (a bacterium) called the pneumococcus (more than one is called pneumococci).
- Pneumococci can cause a number of infections such as:
  - acute ear infection
  - sinus infection
  - pneumonia (lung infection)
  - bacteremia (blood infection)
  - meningitis
  - joint infections
  - bone infections
- Ear infections can lead to deafness.
- Pneumonia, bacteremia, meningitis, and bone and joint infections are very serious illnesses and can kill.
- Meningitis is an infection of the fluid and membranes that cover the brain and spinal cord. Without treatment, all children who get this disease die or suffer damage that lasts the rest of their lives.
- Even with treatment, about 1 in 5 children with pneumococcal meningitis die.
- About 1 in 10 children who survive meningitis have brain damage or are deaf.

How can you tell if you or your child has pneumococcal meningitis?

- The earliest symptoms of meningitis are fever and a significant change in behaviour such as drowsiness, reduced consciousness, irritability, fussiness, and/or agitation.
- Other symptoms include severe headache, vomiting (throwing up), stiff neck, pain on moving head and neck, aches and pains, pain in joints, and convulsions.

How is pneumococcal disease spread?

- Pneumococci are quite common and live in the back of the nose and throat of about 1 in 3 infants, children and adults without causing any illness. These individuals are called carriers.
- The bacteria are fragile and die rapidly outside the body.
- Spread of pneumococci most often involves healthy carriers rather than persons ill with visible disease.
- Spread from an infected person to another person requires close, direct contact, through activities such as kissing, coughing and sneezing.
- It can also be spread through saliva when sharing items such as cigarettes, lipstick, food or drinks, cups, water bottles, cans, drinking straws, toothbrushes, toys, mouthguards and musical instruments with mouthpieces.
- The risk of spread is increased by smoking and by overcrowding.

How common is pneumococcal disease?

- Every year in Canada, about 65 infants less than 2 years of age suffer meningitis; 700 have bacteremia;

2,200 have pneumonia; and 200,000 have an ear infection, all caused by pneumococci.

What can you do to stop the spread of pneumococcal disease?

- Get a pneumococcal shot. Two kinds of pneumococcal vaccine are available.
- One vaccine is not effective in infants and young children, but is very effective in children over age 5, adolescents, and adults. It is used as a routine vaccine in adults age 65 and over to reduce deaths from pneumococcal pneumonia and bacteremia.
- The other vaccine protects against the most common kinds of pneumococci bacteria that cause severe infections in infants.

How do you get the vaccine?

- Both forms of pneumococcal vaccine are given by injection.
- The vaccine for children age 5 and over, adolescents and adults is given as a single shot.

- The schedule for infants and young children appears below.

AGE AT FIRST DOSE	PRIMARY SERIES	BOOSTER DOSE
2 to 6 months	3 doses, 8 weeks apart	1 dose at 12 to 15 months of age
7 to 11 months	2 doses, 8 weeks apart	1 dose at 12 to 15 months of age and at least 4 weeks after last dose of primary series
12 to 23 months	2 doses, 8 weeks apart	None
24 to 59 months	1 dose	None

Who should *not* have the pneumococcal vaccines?

A person who has had a serious allergic reaction after a previous shot of the pneumococcal vaccine should not receive it again.

How safe are the vaccines?

- Both forms of the vaccine are very safe.
- People often have redness, swelling and pain at the place where they got the needle.
- Ask your doctor what you can do to control pain or swelling.

© CPS, December 2002

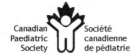

Canadian Paediatric Society

Société canadienne de pédiatrie

100–2204 Walkley Road, Ottawa, ON K1G 4G8 Tel.: (613) 526-9397 Fax: (613) 526-3332 www.caringforkids.cps.ca

Meningococcal Vaccine

What is meningococcal disease?

- Meningococcal disease is caused by a germ (a bacterium) called the meningococcus (more than one is called meningococci).
- Meningococci can cause a very serious infection called meningitis.
- Meningitis is an infection of the fluid and membranes that cover the brain and spinal cord. Without treatment, all children who get this disease will die or suffer damage that lasts the rest of their lives.
- Meningococci can also cause septicemia, a very serious infection of the blood that can kill very rapidly.
- Even with treatment, about 1 in 20 children with meningococcal meningitis will die.
- About 1 in 20 children who survive meningitis will have brain damage.
- Even with treatment, about 1 in 2 children with meningococcal septicemia will die or have permanent damage.

How can you tell if your child has meningococcal meningitis?

- The earliest symptoms of meningitis are fever and a significant change in behaviour such as drowsiness, reduced consciousness, irritability, fussiness and/or agitation.
- Other symptoms include severe headache, vomiting (throwing up), stiff neck, pain on moving head and neck, aches and pains, pain in joints and convulsions.
- About two-thirds of children with meningococcal meningitis have a skin rash consisting of red spots that do not disappear when pressed. The spots may get quite large in a short period of time.

How can you tell if your child has meningococcal septicemia?

- The earliest symptoms of septicemia are fever, aches and pains, joint pain and headache.
- The child gets much sicker very quickly (over a few hours), is drowsy, semi-conscious, irritable or agitated.
- Almost all children with septicemia have a skin rash that starts as red spots. The spots increase in number and size very rapidly over a few hours.
- The illness may progress rapidly and be complicated by low blood pressure (shock), coma, convulsions and severe difficulty breathing.

How is meningococcal disease spread?

- Meningococci are quite common and live in the back of the nose and throat of about 1 in 5 adolescents and adults without causing any illness. These individuals are called "healthy carriers."
- The bacteria are extremely fragile and die rapidly outside the body.
- Spread of meningococci most often involves healthy carriers rather than persons ill with visible disease.
- Spread from an infected person to another person requires close, direct contact, through activities such as kissing, coughing and sneezing.

- It can also be spread through saliva when sharing items such as cigarettes, lipstick, food or drinks, cups, water bottles, cans, drinking straws, toothbrushes, toys, mouth guards and musical instruments with mouthpieces.
- The risk of spread is increased by smoking and by overcrowding.

How common is meningococcal disease?

- About 200 to 400 cases of meningococcal disease occur every year in Canada.
- Group B and group C germs cause most infections in Canada.
- Since 1989, outbreaks of group C disease have occurred among adolescents in many parts of Canada. Such outbreaks usually occur in one or two schools in an area and involve fewer than 5 cases.

What can you do to stop the spread of meningococcal disease?

- Get a meningococcal shot. Two kinds of meningococcal vaccine are available. One is more effective in infants and young children. The other one prevents disease in children age 5 and over, adolescents and adults. Your doctor will know which one to give you or your child.
- Family and household members of a person sick with meningococcal disease are often treated with an antibiotic to stop further spread of the germ within the household.

How do you get the vaccine?

- Both forms of meningococcal vaccine are given by injection.
- The vaccine is given as a single dose.
- Very young infants get 3 shots: one at 2, 4 and 6 months of age. Infants between 4 and 11 months of age receive 2 shots at least 4 weeks apart. Children over 12 months of age get 1 shot.

Who should *not* have the meningococcal vaccines?

A person who has had a serious allergic reaction after a previous shot of the meningococcal vaccine should not receive it again.

How safe are the vaccines?

- Both forms of the vaccine are very safe.
- They often cause redness, swelling and pain at the place where you get the needle.
- Ask your doctor what you can do to control pain or swelling.

© CPS, December 2002

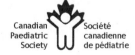

Canadian Paediatric Society   Société canadienne de pédiatrie

100–2204 Walkley Road, Ottawa, ON K1G 4G8 Tel.: (613) 526-9397 Fax: (613) 526-3332 www.caringforkids.cps.ca

Hepatitis B Vaccine

What is hepatitis B?

- It is a disease caused by a virus. A virus is a kind of germ that can make people sick.
- The hepatitis B virus attacks the liver.
- Sometimes, people with hepatitis B do not feel sick at all. But they can still pass the disease on to other people. They are called carriers.
- In other cases, hepatitis B makes people very sick. It can cause serious damage to the liver and long-lasting (or chronic) liver disease. Hepatitis B is one of the main reasons people get liver cancer.
- There is no cure for hepatitis B.

How can you tell if you have hepatitis B?

Go for a blood test at a health clinic or your doctor's office.

How is hepatitis B spread?

It is *not* spread by sneezing, coughing, hugging or using the same dishes, forks or knives.

It spreads from person to person when body fluids are passed between people. The kinds of body fluids that spread hepatitis B are:

- blood;
- breast milk;
- semen (the liquid that comes from a man's penis during sex); and
- fluids in a woman's vagina.

Hepatitis B can be spread in the following ways:

- During sexual activity.
- From sharing needles during drug use.
- From infected needles, for example in a tattoo shop or when you have your ears or other parts of your body pierced.
- From a woman to her baby during birth, pregnancy or breastfeeding.
- From sharing toothbrushes or razors (when blood has been in touch with the toothbrush or razor).

How common is hepatitis B?

- In Canada, there are about 20,000 new cases each year.
- It is most common among young adults. They can get it from having sex without a condom. Sharing needles when they take drugs can spread hepatitis B. So can dirty needles that are used to do a tattoo or pierce ears or other body parts.
- The number of babies born with hepatitis B is lower now than it used to be. This is because pregnant women are being tested for the disease and their babies are given the shot as soon as they are born.
- In other parts of the world, hepatitis B is more common than in Canada. If you travel to China, Southeast Asia or some parts of Africa, you may be at higher risk.

What can you do to stop the spread of hepatitis B?

- Get the hepatitis B shot.
- If you take drugs, don't share needles.
- Always wear a condom when you have sex with someone other than your regular partner.
- If you are pregnant, have a blood test to see if you have hepatitis B. If you have hepatitis B, your baby can start getting the shots to prevent hepatitis B as soon as it is born.
- If you know someone who has hepatitis B, be careful not to touch their blood, if they are bleeding.

How do you get the vaccine?

- A nurse or doctor gives you a needle in your arm or leg. You need 2 or 3 shots to be protected.
- People usually get the shots over 6 months.
- In special cases, the shots may be given more often.

How safe is the vaccine?

- It is one of the safest vaccines used today.
- When you get any vaccine, you may have redness, swelling or pain at the place where you got the needle.
- Ask your doctor what you can take to control pain or swelling.

© CPS, December 2002

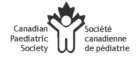

Canadian
Paediatric
Society

Société
canadienne
de pédiatrie

100–2204 Walkley Road, Ottawa, ON K1G 4G8 Tel.: (613) 526-9397 Fax: (613) 526-3332 www.caringforkids.cps.ca

Td (Tetanus and Lower-Dose Diphtheria) Vaccine

If you are between the ages of 14 and 16, you're in for a boost! To be more exact, you have reached the age when you need to have a booster shot for two serious diseases:

1. Tetanus, and
2. Diphtheria.

You probably got needles for these diseases when you were much younger. Those shots protected you for about 10 years. Now, it's time to protect yourself again.

What is tetanus?

- It is also called lockjaw.
- It is caused by germs (bacteria) that live in dirt and dust.
- If tetanus germs get into an open cut on your body, poison from the germs can spread to nerves and then to your muscles. Muscles may lock in one place or go into spasms (get very tight). This is very painful.
- In most cases, the first muscles affected are in the jaw. You may not be able to swallow or open your mouth. This is why tetanus is called lockjaw.
- If the poison gets to the muscles that help you breathe, you can die quickly.
- The main treatment for tetanus is drugs (antibiotics) to kill the germs. You can also get other drugs to control the muscle spasms.

- People who survive tetanus may have long-lasting problems with speech, memory and thinking.
- People who survive can still get tetanus again. For this reason, they should get the vaccine to protect them in the future.

How is tetanus spread?

- It is not spread from person to person. The only way to get it is when dirt or dust that carries germs gets into a cut.

What is diphtheria?

- It is an illness caused by germs (bacteria) that infect the nose, throat or skin.
- It causes serious problems with breathing. It can also cause heart failure and nerve damage that will affect you for the rest of your life.
- Of every 10 people who get diphtheria, 1 will die from it. Babies who get it are even more likely to die.
- There is no good treatment for diphtheria.
- People who survive diphtheria can still get it again. For this reason, they should get the vaccine to protect them in the future.

How is diphtheria spread?

- It is spread by close, direct contact between people. Sneezes or coughs from a person with diphtheria can infect someone who doesn't have the disease.

How safe are the vaccines?

- The tetanus vaccine is one of the safest. Because tetanus germs can be found anywhere, the best way to prevent tetanus is by getting the shot.
- The diphtheria vaccine is very safe. The only reason not to get the shot is if you had trouble breathing or severe swelling of the skin or mouth when you got it before.
- When you get any vaccine, you may have redness, swelling or pain at the place where the needle went in.
- Ask your doctor what you can take to control the pain or swelling.

What is the dTap vaccine?

- Soon, the Td vaccine combined with the adult form of acellular pertussis vaccine will be used routinely for the booster at 14 to 16 years of age rather than Td alone.
- The reason for adding the acellular pertussis vaccine is to boost immunity against pertussis.

- The pertussis vaccine you probably received when you were younger is very effective, but its protection wears off. Many teenagers are susceptible to pertussis.
- Outbreaks of pertussis in junior and senior high schools have become common.

What is pertussis?

- It is an illness caused by germs (bacteria) that get into the throat and lungs.
- Pertussis in teenagers causes a severe cough that lasts 2 to 3 weeks or more.
- Complications of pertussis are rare, but the coughing spells can interfere with sleep and physical activity, and cause loss of time from school and work.

Is the dTap vaccine safe?

- It is a very safe vaccine.
- Reactions after the dTap vaccine are similar to those after Td alone. There is a slight increase in redness and swelling at the place where the needle goes into the skin, but with little or no pain.
- It will protect you against all three diseases.

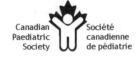

Canadian Paediatric Society   Société canadienne de pédiatrie

100–2204 Walkley Road, Ottawa, ON K1G 4G8 Tel.: (613) 526-9397 Fax: (613) 526-3332 www.caringforkids.cps.ca

Influenza Vaccine

What is influenza?

- Influenza (sometimes called flu) is a virus that causes epidemics of colds, bronchitis (infection of the airways) and pneumonia (infection of the lungs) every year in the late fall or winter.
- The illness caused by influenza virus may be the same as illness caused by a cold virus, but the influenza virus is much more dangerous.
- It can cause severe illness and death.
- Sometimes, you get just a cold with a runny nose, sore throat, cough and fever. But usually, there is also headache, muscle pain and marked loss of energy.
- Complications of influenza include ear infections, bronchitis and pneumonia. Complications are much more common and serious (even fatal) in infants (children under 12 months), persons aged 65 and over, and anyone with chronic heart or lung disease, regardless of age.

Who should have a flu shot?

- Health Canada recommends that healthy adults and their children who want to protect themselves from influenza should receive the vaccine.
- Health Canada also recommends that children who are at high risk from complications from flu should get a flu shot. This means children who:
  - have chronic heart or lung problems (e.g., cystic fibrosis, asthma)
  - have other chronic conditions like immune deficiencies and metabolic diseases
  - have cancer
  - have to take ASA (acetylsalicylic acid or Aspirin) on a daily basis
- Talk to your doctor if you think your child should have a flu shot.

Who should *not* have the influenza vaccine?

You should *not* get a flu shot if you:
- are under 6 months of age;
- have an allergy to eggs;
- are pregnant or breastfeeding; or
- have an allergy to thimerosal (a preservative containing mercury that is used in contact lens solutions and the flu vaccine).

When should you have a flu shot?

Flu shots are usually given from October to mid-November. They provide protection throughout the flu season (October to March).

How safe is the vaccine?

- The vaccine is very safe.

About this information

This fact sheet gives you basic information about the vaccine and the disease it protects against. It should not be used as a substitute for the medical care and advice of your doctor. Treatment can vary based on individual facts and circumstances. Ask your doctor any questions you have about the vaccine *before* your child is vaccinated.

Health care professionals may reproduce these sheets without permission and share them with patients and their families.

© CPS, December 2002

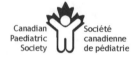

Canadian Paediatric Society

Société canadienne de pédiatrie

100–2204 Walkley Road, Ottawa, ON K1G 4G8 Tel.: (613) 526-9397 Fax: (613) 526-3332 www.caringforkids.cps.ca

Routine childhood immunization schedule

Age	VACCINES*							
	DTaP/IPV	Hib	MMR	VZ	PC	MC	Hep B†	Td/dTap
2 months	X	X			X	X		
4 months	X	X			X	X		
6 months	X	X			X	X		
12 months			X	X	X			
18 months	X	X						
4–6 years	X		X‡					
Pre-teen							X	
14–16 years								X

* DTaP/IPV: diphtheria and tetanus toxoids and acellular pertussis and inactivated polio vaccines

   Hib: *Haemophilus influenzae* type b conjugate vaccine

   MMR: measles, mumps and rubella vaccines

   VZ: varicella (chickenpox) vaccine

   PC: pneumococcal conjugate vaccine

   MC: meningococcal group C conjugate vaccine

   Hep B: hepatitis B vaccine (3 doses in infants and young children; 2 doses in children 11 years of age or older).

   Td or dTap: tetanus and lower-dose diphtheria or tetanus, lower-dose diphtheria and the adult form of acellular pertussis vaccine

† Hepatitis B vaccine is recommended for all newborn infants whose mothers are infected with hepatitis B. Some provinces and territories recommend routine vaccination of all infants in addition to pre-teenage children.

‡ The second dose of MMR is given at 18 months in some provinces and territories.

About this information

This fact sheet gives you basic information about vaccines and the diseases they protect against. It should not be used as a substitute for the medical care and advice of your doctor. Treatment can vary based on individual facts and circumstances. Ask your doctor any questions you have about the vaccine *before* your child is vaccinated.

Health care professionals may reproduce these sheets without permission and share them with patients and their families.

© CPS, December 2002

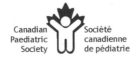

Canadian Paediatric Society   Société canadienne de pédiatrie

100–2204 Walkley Road, Ottawa, ON K1G 4G8 Tel.: (613) 526-9397 Fax: (613) 526-3332 www.caringforkids.cps.ca

Index

A page number in italic indicates that the information is in a Table or Figure on that page.

natural infection 9, 274-75
naturopathy 273, 292
necrotizing fasciitis 16, 237
Neisseria meningitidis 211
Nepal, polio 79
nephritis 257
nerve damage 31
Netherlands
    disease outbreaks 2
    Hib 96
    polio 91-92
neurologic problems 49, 281
New Zealand
    hepatitis B 172
    polio 78-79
    SIDS 291
nurses 15, 17
nutrition 265-66

– O –
oculo-respiratory syndrome 188
OPV *see* oral polio vaccine (OPV)
oral polio vaccine (OPV)
    defined 83
    effectiveness 91-92
    given with measles vaccine 127
    how given 87
    making 85-86
    side effects 88-90, 267-68
orchitis 137, 263
osteomyelitis 99-100
otitis
    from Hib 99, *101*
    from pneumococci 197, 200

– P –
Paediatrics & Child Health 19
Pakistan, polio 79
Pan American Health Organization 16
pancreatitis 137
pandemics 178, 180
Panum, Peter 112
paralysis
    from oral polio vaccine 88
    from polio 81-82, 262
Parents of Kids with Infectious Diseaes 307
Pediatrics 19
pertussis
    cause 53, 55-56
    complications 58-59, *270*
    diagnosis 59
    fact sheet 312-13, 324-25
    history 53-55
    number of cases 54-55, 72, 265, *270*
    outbreaks in other countries 70-74
    seriousness 262, 268, *270*
    spread 57
    symptoms 57-58, *270*
    treatment 59
    vaccination 62-75, 268, *270*, 284-85
    vaccine 60-62, *310*
Peru, polio 79

pneumococcal conjugate vaccine 202-04, 207, 209
pneumococcal disease
    cause 193, 195
    complications 200
    diagnosis 200
    fact sheet 318-19
    history 194
    number of cases 194
    persons at high risk *205*
    seriousness 264, 269
    spread 196
    symptoms 196-200
    treatment 200-201
    vaccination 203-09, 269
    vaccines 194, 201-03, *310*
pneumococcal polysaccharide vaccine 201-02, 204,
    207, 209
pneumonia
    from chickenpox 237, 264
    from group B streptococcus 258
    from Hib 99, *101*, 269
    from influenza 177
    from measles 117, 263
    from pneumococci 198, 269
polio
    cause 77, 79-80
    complications 82, *270*
    diagnosis 82
    eradication campaign 16, 79, 92, 262, 267
    fact sheet 312-13
    history 77-79
    number of cases 78, 265, *270*
    outbreaks in other countries 2, 262
    seriousness 262, *270*
    spread 79-81
    symptoms 81-82, *270*
    treatment 83
    vaccination 87-92, *270*
    vaccines 83-87, *310*
poliovirus 77-80
postherpetic neuralgia 239
post-marketing surveillance 14-18
potency tests 14
pregnancy
    and chickenpox 238, 244
    and hepatitis B 165, 173
    and influenza vaccine 189
    and measles 118, 126
    and mumps 137, 142
    and rubella 145-46, 148, 151, 263, 269
    and rubella vaccine 155, 157-58, 269
production standards 14
provinces and territories, role in vaccine safety 14-15,
    18
public health 15
purified bacterial polysaccharide or complex sugar
    example *10*
    for Hib 104, 267
    for meningococcal disease 219, 267
    for pneumococcal disease 201, 267
    for typhoid fever 253-54